THE DIET SOLUTION

WEIGHT LOSS, WELLNESS, AND THE WORD OF WISDOM

PEGGY J. HUGHES

EAGLE GATE

Library of Congress Cataloging-in-Publication Data

Hughes, Peggy Jordan, 1948–
    The diet solution: weight loss, wellness, and the word of wisdom / Peggy Jordan Hughes.
      p. cm.
    ISBN-10 1-57345-656-X (pbk.)
    ISBN-13 978-1-57345-656-2 (pbk.)
    1. Weight loss   I. Title
RM222.2+
613.7—dc21   00-028809

Printed in the United States of America

10   9   8   7   6   5   4   3

CONTENTS

SECTION FOUR: APPENDIXES

FOREWORD

In more than twenty years as a registered dietician, I have worked with hundreds of people who are trying to manage their weight. For them, a common pitfall is focusing on quick fixes rather than on long-term lifestyle changes. Quick fixes are snazzy, very different from normal eating patterns, and generally successful for only a short time. Lifestyle changes focus on overall health, bring about gradual change, and are intended to last a lifetime.

In *The Diet Solution*, Peggy Hughes focuses on healthy lifestyles. Her book integrates current findings about nutrition and health with scriptural counsel regarding care of the body. While individuals with specific medical conditions need to follow the advice of their physicians and dieticians, the vast majority of people will find sensible, sound guidance about eating and exercise in *The Diet Solution*.

The gift of a mortal body is most precious. Care and keeping of the body is not supposed to be the primary focus of our time and energy—the primary focus should be on relationships with others and accomplishing good works. Without some attention, however, the body will not be healthy enough to allow us to do what we are on earth to do. *The Diet Solution* examines both the spiritual and physical dimensions of life and shows how the physical can support the spiritual. Through practical pointers and concrete examples, Peggy Hughes provides help for those wanting to improve their lifestyles.

—Nora Nyland, Ph.D., R.D.

Acknowledgments

I am grateful to Nora Nyland, a registered dietician and the director of the dietetics program in the Food Science and Nutrition Department at Brigham Young University, for her guidance, suggestions, wisdom, and support in reviewing and consulting on this project.

I would also like to thank Shawn Fluharty for her assistance with the exercise portion of this book. Shawn is finishing her Ph.D. and is an instructor specializing in biomechanics in the physical education department at Brigham Young University. She reviewed the two exercise chapters and let me videotape her doing all the exercises to ensure that the photographs accurately depict how the exercises should be done.

Finally, I would like to thank my daughter Jenny Slingerland, who modeled for the pictures, and Alan Blakely, who photographed them.

Introduction
A SPIRITUAL SOLUTION

It was a cold winter's day in February 1833 when Joseph Smith and other leaders of the Church met in Joseph's Kirtland, Ohio, home to hear instructions on Church doctrine. The windows were shut, and the air was thick with tobacco smoke. Several of the men in the little room were chewing large plugs of tobacco and aiming the brown spittle at brass spittoons.

When the meeting concluded later that day, the air was stale and the floor covered with the men's missed attempts. Joseph's wife, Emma, came in to clean up and was disgusted by the sight and smell. She went to see her husband. I can almost hear her saying, "Who do you expect to clean up this mess?"

The practice had been troubling Joseph for some time as well. He was familiar with verses of scripture that said the body is the temple of God: "Know ye not that ye are the temple of God, and that the Spirit of God dwelleth in you? If any man defile the temple of God, him shall God destroy; for the temple of God is holy, which temple ye are" (1 Corinthians 3:16–17).

Joseph took the matter to the Lord and received the Word of Wisdom, recorded in the Doctrine and Covenants, section 89:[1]

A Word of Wisdom, . . .

Given for a principle with promise, adapted to the capacity of the weak and the weakest of all saints, who are or can be called saints.

Behold, verily, thus saith the Lord unto you: In consequence of evils and designs which do and will exist in the hearts of conspiring men in the last days, I have warned you, and forewarn you, by giving unto you this word of wisdom by revelation—

That inasmuch as any man drinketh wine or strong drink among you, behold it is not good, neither meet in the sight of your Father, only in assembling yourselves together to offer up your sacraments before him.

And, behold, this should be wine, yea, pure wine of the grape of the vine, of your own make.

And, again, strong drinks are not for the belly, but for the washing of your bodies.

And again, tobacco is not for the body, neither for the belly, and is not good for man, but is an herb for bruises and all sick cattle, to be used with judgment and skill.

And again, hot drinks are not for the body or belly.

And again, verily I say unto you, all wholesome herbs God hath ordained for the constitution, nature, and use of man—

Every herb in the season thereof, and every fruit in the season thereof; all these to be used with prudence and thanksgiving.

Yea, flesh also of beasts and of the fowls of the air, I, the Lord, have ordained for the use of man with thanksgiving; nevertheless they are to be used sparingly;

And it is pleasing unto me that they should not be used, only in times of winter, or of cold, or famine.

All grain is ordained for the use of man and of beasts, to be the staff of life, not only for man but for the beasts of the field, and the fowls of heaven, and all wild animals that run or creep on the earth;

And these hath God made for the use of man only in times of famine and excess of hunger.

All grain is good for the food of man; as also the fruit of the vine; that which yieldeth fruit, whether in the ground or above the ground—

Nevertheless, wheat for man, and corn for the ox, and oats for the horse, and rye for the fowls and for swine, and for all beasts of the field, and barley for all useful animals, and for mild drinks, as also other grain.

And all saints who remember to keep and do these sayings, walking in obedience to the commandments, shall receive health in their navel and marrow to their bones;

And shall find wisdom and great treasures of knowledge, even hidden treasures;

And shall run and not be weary, and shall walk and not faint.

And I, the Lord, give unto them a promise, that the destroying angel shall pass by them, as the children of Israel, and not slay them. Amen. [Vv. 3–21]

Simply put, the Word of Wisdom is this:

No	Yes
strong drinks—	*wholesome herbs*—
liquor, wine, beer	includes vegetables
tobacco—	*fruits*—
in any form	especially those in season
hot drinks—	*meats*—
defined as tea	to be used *sparingly*
and coffee	*grains*—
drugs—	especially wheat
except recognized	
medicines (a later	
addition)	

Joseph Smith received the Word of Wisdom long before science testified to the physical dangers of liquor, tobacco, and caffeine. But for those who have observed it through the ensuing decades, its promises have been fulfilled and extended for generations. In recent times studies have shown that Latter-day Saints who live their religion have fewer incidences of cancer and heart disease than the general American population.[2] Seventh-Day Adventists, who practice a dietary code similar to the Word of Wisdom, also have lower rates of cancer and heart disease.[3]

Certainly, following the Word of Wisdom brings profound rewards. You will be healthier if you do so, but you can also be leaner. And, happily, following the Word of Wisdom doesn't mean you have to starve yourself or try the latest fad diet.

---

d i • e t < Gr. *diaita,* way of life, regimen

1. *b)* what a person regularly reads, listens to, does, etc.

2. a regimen of special or limited food and drink, chosen or prescribed for health or to gain or lose weight (*Webster's New World Dictionary*).

Look at the definition of the word *diet.* Typically the word is associated with eating to lose weight. But when we incorporate the Word of Wisdom into our concept of "diet," the definition changes. From the Greek, *diet* is "a way of life," or "a regular routine." That is the intention of the Word of Wisdom and the intention of this book: to help individuals make changes in their ways of life that will have positive effects on their spiritual and temporal well-being.

I have been on many diets over the years. They were all ultimately unsuccessful. Sooner or later, like most people, I always gained back the weight and then some. Several popular diets on the market now stress the consumption of high-protein foods and very few carbohydrates. As I looked at some of the latest crazes, I asked myself, "How is this really going to work and how healthy am I going to be if this diet is contrary to the Word of Wisdom?"

I began studying the Word of Wisdom and reading from the Prophet Brigham Young's discourses on the subject. I then combined the Word of Wisdom and Brigham Young's writings with what I knew about proper nutrition. In doing so I kept in mind that the Word of Wisdom is not just a way of improving our bodies; it is a way of improving our spirits. The Lord told Joseph Smith that "all things unto me are spiritual, and not at any time have I given unto you a law which was temporal" (D&C 29:34). For this reason I felt it was important that my diet, as a way of life, include a spiritual component along with the temporal advice in the Word of Wisdom.

Brigham Young said, "The Lord has planted within us a divinity; and that divine, immortal spirit requires to be fed. Will earthly food answer for that purpose? No; it will only keep this body alive as long as the spirit stays with it, which gives us an opportunity of doing good."[4]

It became clear to me that spiritual nourishment has to be part of healthy living. Therefore, we need to set a spiritual goal as well as a weight goal. I now find that it is easier to eat properly when I realize that I am not dieting to look like a model, but rather because I want to more fully obey the Word of Wisdom and benefit from its promised blessings.

WHAT IS THE DIET SOLUTION?

The Diet Solution is, first, a family-healthy eating plan, combined with aerobic exercises and strength training—all of which can be done at home. The foods emphasized here are those emphasized in the Word of Wisdom—grains, fruits, vegetables, and meat (but only sparingly).

Of course, knowing what to eat is only part of the solution. The real trick is knowing how to incorporate these types of foods into your eating habits. The Diet Solution teaches you the reasons for cutting back on meat consumption and provides ways to use other foods in place of meats.

It is not a fad diet that you will give up on because of unreasonable prohibitions. Some diets require cutting out all sugar—even fresh vegetables, which naturally contain sugar—or overloading on meat or restricting combinations of foods. On one such popular diet, a person would not be able to eat even a sandwich. The Diet Solution uses the foods that most people already eat and are comfortable with.

It is a *solution* because it incorporates Word of Wisdom eating principles with daily exercise and spiritual nourishment. In this book you will find everything you need to get you started on the road to health and fitness. Recipes and tips on meal planning are included. Easy-to-understand nutritional information is provided; and the reasons for eating certain foods and not others are explained. The exercise section of the book contains routines that can be varied weekly and adapted to any fitness level.

Throughout the book are timeless quotes from Brigham Young on proper diet, eating habits, and the need for exercise. He spoke extensively on these subjects, and his admonitions are as valid today as they were then.

The Diet Solution can work for people of all ages because the healthy-eating guidelines of the Word of Wisdom apply to all age groups. Children need to eat better, as do teenagers, middle-agers, and seniors, who often have special nutritional requirements that the Word of Wisdom can address.

But most important, the Diet Solution works because the Word of Wisdom is also about spiritual nourishment and its connection to our physical health and well-being. The success of this dieting solution lies in the empowering reassurance that the Word of Wisdom is "adapted to the capacity of the weak and the weakest of all saints" (D&C 89:3).

In other words, I can do this! And so can you.

SECTION ONE

Healthy Eating

—————————— 1 ——————————

TIPS TO GET YOU STARTED

*"When you find the thinking faculty perfectly active,
in a healthy person, it should put the physical
organization into active operation. . . . In such a
person you will see mental and physical health and
strength combined, in their perfection."*

—*Brigham Young*

A friend and I were talking recently about the popular diet her husband was on. He was losing quite a bit of weight, but was not happy. She told me he was eating a lot of meat, almost to the exclusion of anything else. She said, "One day he looked at this huge steak he was having for breakfast, put his fork down, and declared, 'This isn't following the Word of Wisdom.'"

Another friend's husband told me his wife was having success on her diet with an expensive weight-loss pill, but he was worried about its long-term consequences. He had read about problems with the herb *ephedra*—also known as *ma huang*—a common ingredient in diet pills. In some people it can cause heart trouble and other serious side effects. He wished she would just eat healthier.

The other day I saw a friend whom I hadn't seen for a long time. She was much thinner than I had remembered.

When I asked her how she had lost her weight, she said, "My husband has a new job that takes him away all week, so when he's gone, I just don't eat."

All these experiences occurred after I had begun writing this book and only confirmed why I developed a diet based on the Word of Wisdom in the first place. If my friends continue on their present course, they are not likely to have the kind of health and strength the Lord intended us to have.

Brigham Young said, "To those who observe [the Word of Wisdom] He will give great wisdom and understanding, increasing their health, giving strength and endurance to the faculties of their bodies and minds until they shall be full of years upon the earth. This will be their blessing if they will observe His word with a good and willing heart and in faithfulness before the Lord."[5]

We have been counseled to focus on commandments we are having trouble obeying, and to work on them until we have mastered them. You probably do not have trouble with the no-drinking, no-smoking, no-coffee, and no-tea part of the Word of Wisdom, but do you view the rest as "optional"? The Word of Wisdom is a commandment *in total;* and you should work at obeying it just as you would any other commandment.

Now, what if you cheat as you begin following the Diet Solution? "Repent," and make amends the next meal or the next day. Do not feel like you are a failure and therefore go back to your old habits. Just start over. Remember, even the weakest of us can do it.

To begin with, here are some pointers to help you get started. Later in the book we'll look at them in more detail.

• *Don't count calories or fat grams.* It is not necessary if you are following the eating plan. In the menu-planning and recipe sections, some fat and calorie information may be given, but only to give you an idea of what you're eating.

• *Have your dessert.* If you are like me, you *need* desserts. Try limiting yourself to *one* dessert a week. It will be something to look forward to, and if you are eating out that week, it would make sense to make that day your dessert day. You do not have to punish yourself if you have more than that, but don't go overboard! Even with desserts there are choices that are more healthy than others. Baked apples, rice pudding, oatmeal cookies with raisins, and fig bars provide some fiber. Whenever Brigham Young traveled throughout the Mormon settlements, the people were anxious to put on their finest meals for him. He told them: "Give me a piece of Johnny-cake; I would rather have it than their pies and tarts and sweet meats. Let me have something that will sustain nature and leave my stomach and whole system clear to receive the Spirit of the Lord and be free from headache and pains of every kind."[6] I've included a pioneer Johnny-cake recipe for you to try.

• *Eat slowly.* It takes time for the brain to get the signal that the stomach is full. Eating slowly will help. If you are still hungry after your meal, leave the table and wait awhile. Chances are the feeling that you need to eat more will pass.

• *Eat often.* Try having several small meals instead of three big meals a day. Research shows you'll burn more calories and keep your blood-sugar levels more even. Blood-sugar levels have a lot to do with hunger pangs, sugar cravings, and how tired you feel. Experts say that after a big meal insulin levels rise and fat may be stored instead of burned.

If you work away from home, keep some snacks in your purse or desk drawer. Snacks might include whole-wheat crackers, graham crackers, raisins, an apple, carrots, celery with a skiff of peanut butter, even a *few* nuts—especially almonds, which are high in vitamin E. But remember, don't eat your snacks *and* three big meals. Those meals will have to be smaller.

• *Pack a snack.* Take something nutritious with you when friends or family want to go get a treat—an apple or banana, for example. Eating is a social experience. You won't be able to just sit there and watch everyone else eat without giving in to the treats yourself. If you have some food with you, you won't miss out on the fun. You could make this outing your weekly dessert event if you are really feeling left out. But I've found that as long as I'm eating *something* I'm happy.

• *Drink lots of water.* Eight glasses of water a day sounds like a lot, and it may take time to work up to that much. I have found it helps if I dress up my water with a slice of lemon or lime and put it in a pretty glass. Substitute the can of soda you keep at your desk with a jug of water. Why waste 150 calories on a can of soda? That can of cola contains about nine teaspoons of sugar! To work it off, you would have to run one and one-half miles.

• *Eat out less often.* My family was in the habit of eating out whenever I didn't feel like cooking, which happened a lot. In addition, we also headed for a fast-food restaurant every Saturday for lunch. Whenever we went for a day's drive we always stopped at a restaurant to eat. Finally I said, "enough." We now eat out one dinner per month and one fast-food lunch per month. Sometimes we skip the monthly dinner out entirely. We have saved a considerable amount of money over the past two years, and I feel that we are doing better at following the counsel to live providently.

If you work and tend to go out for lunch every day, try to cut back. You might try asking out a friend for a healthy breakfast instead, and then have a lighter lunch. Ask your friend out for a walk during the lunch hour. Pack your own lunch and bring it along. That way, you control what you eat.

- *Exercise.* Sorry, but there is no escaping exercise if you want to be healthy and lose weight. Brigham Young said, "As for health, it is far healthier to walk than to ride, and better every way for the people" and, "My mind becomes tired, and perhaps some of yours do. If so, go and exercise your bodies."[7]

- *Rethink meat.* There is quite a bit of detail later in the book, but at this point let's just say that you may need to change your relationship with meat. I know it may go against your families' eating habits, but the Word of Wisdom is very clear on this point: we are to use meat "sparingly." (Note that it does not say we are to forgo meat entirely.)

- *Avoid "Sunday dinner" overeating.* Sunday dinner was always a big event at my house when I was growing up. Often we invited over friends from church. Mom spent hours in the kitchen. There were always lots of meat and mashed potatoes and gravy and yummy desserts. Who could help but overeat? My father and brothers would always lie on the floor for a nap after the huge meal. I think it was because they couldn't move. If the purpose of the Sunday meal is together time, it can be accomplished with simpler fare, and you'll be doing a better job of keeping the Sabbath day holy.

- *Turn off the television.* "Cease to be idle" (D&C 88:124).

- *Smile.* You will look younger and healthier. Scientists say that smiling can lower your blood pressure. Smiling also prompts your body to release endorphins, which make you feel better. Remember, "A merry heart doeth good like a medicine: but a broken spirit drieth the bones" (Proverbs 17:22).

- *Practice visualization.* It works for some people and might help you. Picture yourself wearing clothes you haven't been able to fit into for the last couple of years.

Imagine yourself at a party, but instead of hovering over the food, see yourself taking small portions and spending your time socializing. During the day, before you go out to dinner, visualize yourself ordering a healthy meal and saying "no" to dessert.

• *Don't focus on one day's food intake.* One day is not going to make or break a diet. It is the pattern of your eating that counts.

• *Don't try miracle diets.* Whenever you are tempted to try one of the latest miracle diets, ask yourself, "Is this how I want to eat the rest of my life?" If not, don't go on it. These diets may have temporary success, but when you go off them and resume your normal eating habits you will likely gain back your weight. Ask yourself the same question if you are about to go on a diet pill or appetite suppressant. "Do I want to stay on these pills the rest of my life?" Once you stop taking the pills, your appetite will go back to normal and you will likely regain the weight.

• *Eat at least one meal a day at home as a family.* You'll all eat healthier. Moms no longer control the nutrition of children's meals, especially once they become teenagers. Malls, fast-food restaurants, even gas stations are feeding our children, and what they're eating is not good. Be creative. My sister, who has teenage sons, makes breakfast the family meal. Everyone is up early for school and work, but she is up even earlier, fixing a nutritious breakfast for everyone. They have prayer and scripture study around the family table. Do what works for you.

• *Pray for help.* Your health is not a trivial matter. It is critical to you and your family. You can expect the Lord's help on something as important as this. I know a woman who has been very overweight all her life. I saw her the other day and I didn't recognize her. She told me it was prayer that finally worked for her.

2

WHY THE DIET SOLUTION WORKS

*"A thorough reformation is needed in regard
to our eating and drinking, and on this point
I will freely express myself, and shall be glad if
the people will hear, believe and obey."*

—Brigham Young

It was Brigham Young's intent for us to live a long, healthy, and purposeful life. He said: "Then let us seek to extend the present life to the uttermost, by observing every law of health, and by properly balancing labor, study, rest, and recreation, and thus prepare for a better life. Let us teach these principles to our children, that, in the morning of their days, they may be taught to lay the foundation of health and strength and constitution and power of life in their bodies."[8]

Over the years countless books have been written promoting weight loss and health, with little attention being given to the balance spoken of by Brigham Young. At my local bookstore, I counted ten shelves devoted to diet books.

In 1998, *Consumer Reports* asked a panel of doctors and nutritionists to rate the most popular diet books on the market. None of the diets in these books fared well overall in the ratings, except one, which the panelists agreed was too hard to stick to. The experts also concluded that none of the diets was successful at keeping off the weight permanently and that some of the diets were unsafe.[9]

Nutritionists and government health experts roundly criticize one current fad diet—which is low in carbohydrates and high in protein and fat—as unhealthy and potentially dangerous. Carbohydrates should be an essential part of your diet. A lot of protein, especially in the form of meat, is not essential; and too much is undesirable. The Word of Wisdom is clear on this point. What is good about carbohydrates? The energy you need for everything you do comes mostly from carbohydrates. Important vitamins, minerals, and fiber come from carbohydrates. Carbohydrates are either complex, like fruits, vegetables, and grains; or simple, like sugar. Simple carbohydrates tend to be easily broken down by digestion. Complex carbohydrates are molecular chains made up of many simple sugars. They are not broken down as quickly as simple carbohydrates. Does it make any sense to drastically cut your consumption of healthy fruits and vegetables and grains? A diet of whole grains has more fiber than a diet of pasta and white bread, even though both are carbohydrates.

There is such a variety of diets being promoted by celebrities and doctors that it is no wonder people are confused. Fortunately, the Word of Wisdom is as valuable today as when it was first given in 1833.

The best way to lose weight, keep it off, and be healthy is to obey the Word of Wisdom. If we followed it as we should, there *would* be a "thorough reformation." "This Word of Wisdom, which has been supposed to have become stale, and not in force, is like all the counsels of God, in force as much today as it ever was. There is life, everlasting life in it—the life which now is and the life which is to come."[10]

WEIGHT LOSS

We are spending more time preoccupied with our looks and weight and more time and money on diets and diet books, and yet we are still getting heavier. The October 1999 *New England Journal of Medicine* published a study by the American Cancer Society, which said, in part, that 55 percent of American adults are now overweight.[11] *JAMA*, in October 1999, published the results of a study conducted by the Centers for Disease Control and Prevention in Atlanta, Georgia, which said the number of obese people rose from 12 percent of the total population in 1991 to 17.9 percent in 1998.[12]

The health consequences of being overweight are significant. These include an increased risk of heart disease, stroke, high blood pressure, diabetes, osteoarthritis, gallstones, and some forms of cancer.

Before going on a diet, *always* consult with your doctor. You may already be at a healthy weight for your age and body type. Even so, if you are like most people, you still need to improve what you eat. A pinch test, body-fat ratio data, and other charts can help you and your doctor determine if you need to lose weight.

If you diet unnecessarily because you think you need to lose five pounds in order to "look good," you may end up weighing more, not less. Spend more time concentrating on being healthy and doing good works, and less time worrying about whether you are thin. Eating the right foods, getting the right amount of exercise, and maintaining a healthy weight will do wonders for your appearance. Keep in mind that it is possible to be thin and not "look good."

The Food and Drug Administration (FDA) reports that more than eight million Americans a year enroll in weight-loss programs. This number does not include all those who go on diets on their own. Relatively few of the people in programs are successful in keeping off their weight.[13]

The FDA warns consumers to be skeptical of diet claims that use words such as *easy, effortless, guaranteed, miraculous, magical, new discovery, mysterious, exotic, ancient, secret,* or *exclusive.* You should also watch out for diet patches, starch blockers, fat blockers, magnet diet pills, glucomannan (a plant root), bulk fillers, guar gum, and spirulina, a blue-green algae.[14]

Not surprisingly, we are also warned against weight-loss earrings, appetite-suppressing eyeglasses, and electrical muscle stimulators (used for weight loss).[15] What this proves is that people are going to almost any length and expense to lose weight, even if it is only temporary.

If you have been on diets in the past and are back to your old weight, or even heavier, ask yourself why the other diets failed. Don't say, "I couldn't stick to it, I wasn't committed enough." Question instead why you could not stick with it. Think about the diet regimen itself, not your own failings. You will probably realize that the diet you were on was one of the crazes sweeping the country at the time. It was either too low in calories or too restrictive in its food choices, or it required you to do mathematics every time you took a bite. For whatever reason, it was not sensible, and your body knew it. (A word about diet drinks, or meal-replacement drinks as they are sometimes called: I do not think they are a good way to lose weight. You need to know how to eat real food—the right kinds in the right amounts. Besides, they are full of sugar. For example, Slim Fast contains 17 grams of sugar in one serving. Having said that, I need to add that once in a while I still have a Slim Fast if I am rushing out the door and I am going to be gone through lunchtime. It keeps me from stopping at a fast-food restaurant and having a hamburger. Then when I get home I have a piece of fruit or carrots.)

"Yo-yo" dieting can be one of your worst enemies. Going on and off diets can make your body resist losing weight. In desperation, some people eat so little, sometimes 800 calories or less, that they force their metabolism so low they can't lose weight. I know; I've tried it. I wouldn't believe a nutritionist who once told me that I needed more calories to get my metabolism in balance. Some low-calorie diets simply do not provide enough nutrition. They also cause you to lose lean muscle mass as well as fat. Then, when you gain back the weight, it is in the form of fat. With less muscle to burn the increased amount of fat, your ability to burn calories is reduced, and you gain more weight.

On most of my diets over the years all I thought about was food. I would look at my diet constantly to see what and when I could eat next. This obsession, caused by the character of an unrealistic diet, makes dieters "crazy," until we break down, cheat, and then loathe ourselves for our "lack of self-control." The more you have to "do" and the more you have to change your lifestyle to an extreme degree, the more likely the diet will not succeed.

Another way to insure that you won't make it is to deny yourself everything you've always enjoyed. You are not an alcoholic who has to swear off liquor entirely. You just have to eat your favorite fattening foods less often and eat them in smaller portions. If you love coconut cream pie, don't say you'll never eat it again as long as you live. Just say, " I will have only a small slice." Furthermore, your diet is not going to suffer irreparable harm if you eat one more dessert than suggested in the week. Add some extra exercise instead of eating less than you should the next day, or giving up entirely. Don't get the idea, however, that "anything goes" with the Diet Solution. If you do, you won't take it seriously. For example, I like to put a *little* butter and brown sugar on my banana squash. You do not have to apply the same reasoning to putting hot fudge sauce on ice cream.

Here is how I finally got serious about dieting correctly. I had to go to my doctor for some routine tests. The nurse wanted to weigh me. I said, "OK, but don't tell me what it says." I stepped on the scale, and the nurse said, "Close your eyes." I did, but I could hear her moving the weights on the scale farther and farther to the right.

Afterwards, the nurse went to the person who was recording the data and whispered, "She doesn't want to know." The person replied, "Ignorance is bliss." Perhaps, but bad health isn't bliss, and I knew I had to do something. For one thing, as an older mom with a young son I not only wanted to be around to see him grow up, but I also wanted to be able to keep up with him and participate with him in his activities.

Let's start out right this time. If you say, "I'm going to lose X pounds by Memorial Day when the pool opens," and you haven't, you are going to be miserable all summer. Instead, determine how much weight you want to lose. Assume a two-pound loss per week, if you are exercising. More than two pounds is water loss and is temporary. Remember, *the faster you lose your weight, the more likely you are to regain it.* Experts say two pounds is the most to expect and still stay healthy. Say you want to lose thirty pounds; at two pounds per week it will take you fifteen weeks. This will give you a target date. Maybe Memorial Day isn't realistic, but whatever the date turns out to be, plan a celebration or a reward, such as a new outfit.

Weigh yourself once a week to check on your two-pound goal. If you need to, increase your exercise, but don't cut back on your food, assuming you are eating as you should. Even so, your body chemistry may allow you to shed only one pound a week. That's OK. If you are making progress and maintaining your healthy eating and exercise plan, you can still enjoy your summer, even if the target date slips.

Now, decide to be healthy, and then ask Heavenly Father to help. Get support from friends or family. You might want to try the Diet Solution with a friend. Have someone to call and talk to who can encourage you.

If you are about to put something in your mouth that is high in calories or fat, ask yourself, "Why am I eating this? Am I actually hungry, or am I bored, tired, mad, excited, or procrastinating? If so, will eating help? What can I do instead?"

Get up and fold the clothes, or walk around the block, or phone a friend, or walk to the water cooler. If you really are hungry, get the peanut butter crackers and have one.

Always have the right foods on hand and, if possible, in view. You'll be less likely to reach for something less healthy if the right food is staring you in the face. Put tempting foods out of sight or get rid of them.

Smaller portions mean fewer calories and less fat. You will gain weight even on low-calorie food if you eat too much of it. One-half cup—about a handful—is a serving size for most foods. At first, measure out a half-cup portion of peas, cooked rice, mashed potatoes, and so on, just so you can see how much it is. You don't have to do this at each meal, just often enough to fix in your mind the correct amount. Some of the menus I suggest later in the book may call for a one-cup portion of a certain food. Keep in mind that in most cases this would count as two servings.

Brigham Young said, " . . . where food is partaken of chiefly to gratify the pleasurable sensation derived from eating, disease is engendered, and true misery springs out of this unwise gratification. Some healthy, strong-constituted persons can eat large quantities of food with apparent impunity; but, in so doing, the tax they place upon their systems will ultimately bring disease and death." He also said, "Indulgence of appetite is not worthy."[16]

Eating out doesn't have to be a problem. For one thing, you are going to try to eat out less often. That will make things easier. Overeating at restaurants can be inevitable, because of the large servings, but you *can* control your portion sizes. Many restaurants serve you twice what your serving should be, so count on leaving with a doggie bag.

One of my favorite dishes is blackened salmon. At one restaurant I go to, the salmon is served as a ten-ounce portion. Three to four ounces is sufficient, even if it is salmon.

You can overeat on healthy foods, and that is not healthy, nor is it being moderate in all things.

Be choosy about where you eat. The House of Fries is not a good bet.

Some restaurants provide healthier menus than others do, or at least they have a menu you can work your way around. Often the restaurant's chef can accommodate you if you ask. If in doubt, call ahead. Ask if the restaurant offers entrees that are steamed, broiled, baked, or poached. Order a salad as the appetizer. This will help fill you up—just watch the dressings. Always ask for the dressing on the side, and choose the non-creamy type most often. You can also order an appetizer as the main meal and ask for a side of rice or potatoes and vegetables. Salad bars can be deceiving. Coleslaw, cheese, macaroni salad, potato salad, bacon bits, and croutons can load on the fat. Three-bean salad is high in fat. Share a dessert. Don't offset your efforts by ordering soft drinks. Drink water.

Some fast-food restaurants offer baked potatoes. Have one, but with a skiff of butter and the broccoli, if available. Skip the sauces. Pick chicken or fish instead of beef on your taco or sandwich. They are lower in fat. But if the chicken or fish is breaded and deep-fried, you are better off with the beef. If you are dying for a hamburger, get a kid-sized one without the cheese and skip the fries. A plain hamburger has one-half the fat of a bacon cheeseburger. Now, what if you just reach over and have a few of your friend's fries? Those 14 fries just added 225 calories and 11 grams of fat to your waistline.

Water, Water, Water. "It is difficult to find anything more healthy to drink than good cold water. . . . This is the beverage we should drink. It should be our drink at all times," Brigham Young said.[17] Water is an essential nutrient. Its most well-known functions are transporting nutrients to the cells, washing wastes out of the body, and regulating our body temperature through the evaporation of sweat. Water is not just a thirst quencher. In fact, if you drink water only when you are thirsty (and many of us turn to something else), you may still not be getting enough. The advice to drink eight glasses of water a day has been around for a long time and it is still valid. This amount insures you are getting the water you need. Of course, if you are exercising or working in a hot climate you will need to replenish the increased loss of water from your body.

Juices are fine for part of your daily fluid needs because they are made mostly of water and do contain vitamins, but they can also contain a lot of calories. Water is calorie free. Caffeinated drinks, such as cola, are diuretics, meaning they cause you to lose water. You will need to drink more water to compensate. To keep your skin hydrated in dry climates, including on airplanes, drink lots of water. A glass of water can sometimes take the edge off a food craving, although food cravings are not likely to occur if you follow the healthy eating habits recommended in the Diet Solution. Keep a carafe of cold water on your desk, or a jug of water in the refrigerator.

A word about calories. One pound of fat is equal to 3,500 calories. If you eat 500 extra calories per day, you will gain one pound per week. That may sound extreme, but what about 250 extra calories per day, or one pound every two weeks? One extra slice of bread a day could mean an extra ten to twelve pounds a year.

Calorie counting has gone in and out of favor in the dieting world. Two decades ago it seemed to be all that mattered. Then we were told calories did not count; it was fat grams that mattered. So we all ignored calories and started counting fat grams. The problem with this approach was that we started eating a lot of high-calorie foods, provided the fat content was low. Now we know that calories do count, but some calories are more fattening than others.

Fatty foods are more easily converted to stored fat than lower-fat foods.

Although you do not have to count calories to make the Diet Solution work, you need to understand one basic concept that will help you maintain a desirable weight: energy balance. If you eat more calories than your body needs to perform its activities, your body will *store* the calories as fat, and you will gain weight. If you do not eat enough calories to supply your body's needs, or if you exercise, thereby increasing your body's energy needs, your body will *use* stored fat and you will lose weight. Too few calories taken in will also cause your body to use muscle tissue for fuel, and you don't want that. The healthiest approach to weight loss is a combination of less food and more exercise. When you have reached your desirable weight and you want to maintain it, think energy balance. In other words, keep up the exercise and eat sensibly so that you are eating enough to make up for the energy you are expending.

Starting from where you are. Some years ago, my sister, who was in nursing school, asked me to keep a food diary for a week as part of a class project. I returned to her something that looked like this:

Breakfast: Coke, Snickers candy bar
Lunch: chocolate shake, hamburger, fries
Dinner: skipped

For a long time I was able to keep up this kind of eating without serious consequences or weight gain. But I was laying a foundation of poor eating habits and sluggish metabolism that would haunt me in later years.

You do not have to keep a food diary with the Diet Solution, but you should think about the kinds of foods you *usually* eat, and if it's helpful, list them. Look the list over with a critical eye. If you are having dessert once a day; regularly eating fatty meats like hot dogs, ribs, pork chops, and hamburgers; and if you are frequently eating fried foods, salad dressings, cheese, and ice cream, you are due for a change. If your regular snacks are chips, candy, and soda pop you are due for a change.

The "Dietary Guidelines for Americans," developed by the United States Department of Agriculture (USDA) and the U.S. Department of Health and Human Services (HHS), provide a good starting point for analyzing our eating habits. They are also very compatible with the Word of Wisdom. Here is a summary:

• Eat a variety of foods to get the energy, protein, vitamins, minerals, and fiber you need for good health.

• Balance the food you eat with physical activity and maintain or improve your weight to reduce your chances of having high blood pressure, heart disease, a stroke, certain cancers, and the most common kind of diabetes.

• Choose a diet with plenty of grain products, vegetables, and fruits. These provide needed vitamins, minerals, fiber, and complex carbohydrates and can help lower your fat intake.

• Choose a diet low in fat, saturated fat, and cholesterol to reduce your risk of heart attack and certain types of cancer and to help you maintain a healthy weight.

• Choose a diet moderate in sugars. A diet with lots of sugars has too many calories and too few nutrients for most people and can contribute to tooth decay.

• Choose a diet moderate in salt and sodium to help reduce your risk of high blood pressure.[18]

The Food Guide Pyramid, also created by the USDA and HHS, forms the basis of the Diet Solution because its guidelines are similar to those in the Word of Wisdom, with a few exceptions. One is the meat group. I have altered this portion of the pyramid so that more meat substitutes are suggested. We do not need meat every day. What we need are the proteins, vitamins, and minerals found in meat products, and these can come from other sources, such as dried beans, eggs, and nuts. (I have included in Appendix K the Vegetarian Food Pyramid from the Seventh-Day Adventist Dietetic Association. This guide is helpful because it contains a meat-alternative group.) Most people do not regard eggs, beans, fish, and nuts as substitutes for meat and do not know how to use them. The Diet Solution will help you with this. I also suggest that you eat more than the minimum serving of vegetables recommended and that you choose more whole-grain products from the Bread, Cereal, Rice, and Pasta Group. The pyramid shows the number of servings for each food group. Following is the Food Guide Pyramid in its original form.[19]

USDA Food Guide Pyramid
A Guide to Daily Food Choices

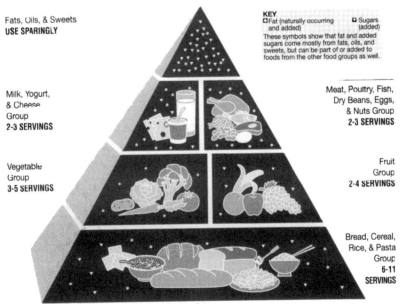

Fats, Oils, & Sweets
USE SPARINGLY

KEY
☐ Fat (naturally occurring and added)   ☐ Sugars (added)
These symbols show that fat and added sugars come mostly from fats, oils, and sweets, but can be part of or added to foods from the other food groups as well.

Milk, Yogurt, & Cheese Group
2-3 SERVINGS

Meat, Poultry, Fish, Dry Beans, Eggs, & Nuts Group
2-3 SERVINGS

Vegetable Group
3-5 SERVINGS

Fruit Group
2-4 SERVINGS

Bread, Cereal, Rice, & Pasta Group
6-11 SERVINGS

SOURCE: U.S. Department of Agriculture/U.S. Department of Health and Human Services.

Here is an example of how you can make the Food Guide Pyramid more closely correspond to the Word of Wisdom. You will be adjusting the food choices and the number of servings, depending on the calorie level you need in the different phases of the Diet Solution (phases and calorie levels will be discussed later).

The Diet Solution Pyramid
Modifying the Food Guide Pyramid

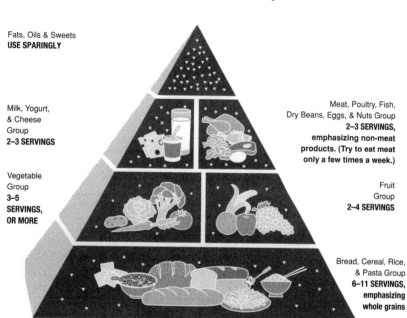

Fats, Oils & Sweets
USE SPARINGLY

Milk, Yogurt,
& Cheese
Group
2–3 SERVINGS

Meat, Poultry, Fish,
Dry Beans, Eggs, & Nuts Group
2–3 SERVINGS,
emphasizing non-meat
products. (Try to eat meat
only a few times a week.)

Vegetable
Group
**3–5
SERVINGS,
OR MORE**

Fruit
Group
2–4 SERVINGS

Bread, Cereal, Rice,
& Pasta Group
6–11 SERVINGS,
emphasizing
whole grains

WHAT COUNTS AS ONE SERVING?

Knowing how much to eat is as important as knowing what to eat when it comes to weight control. Each of the foods listed on the next page counts as one serving in the specified food group.

Bread, Cereal, Rice, & Pasta Group

1 slice of bread
½ English muffin
1 ounce ready-to-eat cereal
½ cup cooked cereal, rice, or pasta
1 tortilla
1 pancake
½ roll, bagel

Vegetable Group

1 cup raw leafy vegetables
½ cup other vegetables—cooked or raw
¾ cup vegetable juice

Fruit Group

1 medium apple, banana, or other fruit
½ cup chopped, cooked, or canned fruit
¾ cup fruit juice
¼ cup dried fruit

Milk, Yogurt, & Cheese Group

1 cup of milk or yogurt
1½ ounces natural cheese
2 ounces processed cheese

Meat, Poultry, Fish, Dry Beans, Eggs, & Nuts Group

2–3 ounces cooked fish, *lean* meat, or poultry (*use sparingly*—3 ounces is about the size of a deck of cards)
1 cup cooked dry beans or 2 eggs each counts as 1 serving of meat
4 tablespoons peanut butter or ½ cup nuts each counts as 1 serving of meat

Usually we eat combinations of these foods, as in casseroles, pizzas, omelets, stir-fry, and so forth. When this is the case, the foods fit in several different parts of the pyramid. Count them as full or partial servings, depending on the amount used in the dish.

Now, with what you know so far, you can start making a few better food choices. You have probably heard the saying: "Don't waste good calories on 'bad' food." But many experts are now saying there is no such thing as a "bad" food (although I am not so sure about fried pork rinds). A "bad" food is just a food you should not eat as often. Choose *more* often lower-calorie, lower-fat foods and prepare your food with less fat. You can take a 100-calorie baked potato and turn it into a 200- or 300-calorie baked potato just by adding one or two tablespoons of butter. A *little* butter or margarine is fine. Baking, grilling, or broiling foods instead of frying them can substantially cut the amount of fat in your diet, as can using skim milk, trimming the fat off meats, and taking the skin off poultry before cooking. So does this mean you can never again have a piece of fried chicken? Of course not. But try eating a smaller amount of fried chicken and only occasionally. Fat and cholesterol will be discussed in more detail in Chapter 10, but on the next page is a chart that will help when you are making food choices.[20]

As you can see, some very simple changes in food choices can make a major difference in your weight. One problem with fixed diet plans is that we do not learn how to make the right food choices once we are on our own. Knowing what foods to choose and why frees us to be able to eat the right foods wherever we are.

Meal Comparison

Higher-Fat Meal	Lower-Fat Meal
Fried chicken (thigh and drumstick) . . . . . 3 tsp. of fat	Baked chicken (thigh and drumstick) . . . . 2 tsp. of fat
French Fries, 10 strips 2 tsp. of fat	Baked potato, 1 med. . . . . . . no fat
	Margarine, 1 tsp. . . . . . . 1 tsp. of fat
Green beans, $^1/_2$ c. and butter, 1 tsp. . . . 1 tsp. of fat	Green beans, $^1/_2$ c. plain . . . . no fat
Whole milk, 1 c. . . . . . . 2 tsp. of fat	2% lowfat milk, 1 c. . . 1 tsp. of fat
Apple pie, 1 slice . . . . . 3 tsp. of fat	Baked apple, 1 lrg. . . . . no fat
Total = 11 tsp. of fat	**Total = 4 tsp. of fat**

3

HOW THE DIET SOLUTION WORKS

"We came to this earth that we might have a body and present it pure before God in the celestial kingdom. The great principle of happiness consists in having a body."

—*Joseph Smith Jr.*

Not all food, even "good" food, is equally nutritious. Some foods pack more nutrients per calorie than others. To illustrate this concept, the Oregon Dairy Council has devised what it calls "Pyramid Plus." Pyramid Plus breaks down the USDA's Food Guide Pyramid to show consumers which foods in each group are the healthiest. Four-star foods are the most nutrient-rich and are often the lowest in calories and fat. One-star foods have less nutrition per calorie. They are not "bad" foods, just foods to choose less often. (Most of the foods in the vegetable and fruit groups are still low in calories and low in fat, regardless of their rating.) The following chart summarizes the Dairy Council's Pyramid Plus. Nutrients are listed under each food group heading.[21]

Breads & Cereals
Supplies: Fiber, Complex Carbohydrates, thiamin, iron, niacin

★★★★ (Most Nutrients)	★★★	★★	★ (Fewest Nutrients)
Barley	Brown rice	Flour tortillas	Cornbread
Bulgur	Bran muffin	Bagel	Fruit or nut bread
Bran or whole-grain cereals	Whole-grain crackers	Enriched breads	Biscuit
Popcorn (air-popped or light microwave)	Soft pretzel	Enriched rice	Stuffing
Whole-grain breads	English muffin	Pancakes	Croissant
Oatmeal	Enriched pasta	Waffles	
Whole-grain pasta	Popcorn (oil-popped)	Graham crackers	
Corn or whole-wheat tortillas		Saltines	
		Sweetened cereal	
		Dry pretzels	

Vegetables
Supplies: Folic Acid, Vitamins A and C, fiber

★★★★ (Most Nutrients)	★★★	★★	★ (Fewest Nutrients)
Red and green bell peppers	Cabbage	Beets	Eggplant
Mustard greens	Chard	Cucumber	Corn
Bok choy	Asparagus	Celery	Avocado
Spinach	Kale	Jicama	Potato
Leaf lettuce	Vegetable juice	Artichoke	
Broccoli	Brussels sprouts	Peas	
Carrots	Salsa	Mushrooms	
Cauliflower	Iceberg lettuce		
	Sweet potato		
	Tomato		
	Snow peas		
	Zucchini		
	Okra		
	Winter squash		
	Green beans		

Fruits
Supplies: Folic Acid, Vitamins A and C, fiber

★★★★ (Most Nutrients)	★★★	★★	★ (Fewest Nutrients)
Papaya	Honeydew	Peach	Pear
Strawberries	Raspberries	Nectarine	Apple
Kiwi	Apricots	Banana	Dried fruit
Orange	Rhubarb	Plum	Grapes
Grapefruit	Pineapple	Cherries	Raisins
Orange juice	Watermelon	Frozen fruit	
Cantaloupe	Pineapple juice	juice bar	
Mandarin	Blueberries	Canned fruit	
oranges			
Mango			

Milk & Milk Products
Supplies: Calcium, riboflavin, protein

★★★★ (Most Nutrients)	★★★	★★	★ (Fewest Nutrients)
Nonfat plain	Part-skim ricotta	Pudding	Milkshake
yogurt	cheese	Custard	Cottage cheese
Nonfat milk	Whole milk	Low-fat frozen	Ice cream
Nonfat cream	Regular-fat	yogurt	Nonfat sour
cheese	cheese	Light ice cream	cream
Nonfat fruit	Low-fat choco-		
yogurt	late milk (1%)		
Low-fat milk	Low-fat fruit		
(1%)	yogurt		
Buttermilk	Nonfat frozen		
Low-fat cheese	yogurt		
Reduced fat			
milk (2%)			

Meat & Meat Alternatives
Supplies: Iron, Protein, niacin, thiamin, zinc, B₁₂

★★★★ (Most Nutrients)	★★★	★★	★ (Fewest Nutrients)
Fish	Beef (rib, chuck, flank, and ground)	Hot dogs	Peanut butter
Shellfish		Pork sausage	Bologna
Poultry (light meat, skinless)	Egg substitute	Chicken nuggets	
Turkey ham	Ham (lean)	Fish sticks	
Beef (round and sirloin)	Tofu	Nuts and seeds	
Pork (tenderloin)	Veal and lamb (leg and loin)		
Veal (leg and shoulder)	Poultry (dark meat with skin)		
Lentils	Pork (loin chop and rib)		
	Canadian bacon		
	Poultry sausage		
	Dried beans and peas		
	Eggs		

Source: Nutrition Education Services/Oregon Dairy Council.

If you are using the Diet Solution to lose weight, do the following, and remember that calorie levels are approximate. (If you are tall or very active, begin at a higher calorie range.)

You should not eat fewer than 1,200 calories a day, but you may, in time, be able to maintain your desired weight while eating more than 1,800 calories a day. You will probably have to adjust how much you eat until you find the calorie level that is right for you. The number of calories you can eat to lose weight is highly individual. It will vary according to your age, height, level of activity, and heredity. You have probably noticed that serving sizes on Nutrition

Facts labels are based on a 2,000-calorie diet. This does not necessarily apply to you. The 2,000-calorie diet is based on what a "typical" woman eats who is not trying to lose weight. Eating 2,000 calories a day, even at the maintenance phase of this diet, may be too high if you are older or not particularly active. The calorie ranges and serving recommendations given in the Diet Solution are designed primarily for women. Most teenagers and men need more calories and will have to make adjustments to the Diet Solution as needed.

Because each person's body is different and may require eating more or less, you might want to consider talking to a registered dietician. Most hospitals and wellness centers have one on staff. You can also find a registered dietician in your area by calling the American Dietetic Association at 1-800-366-1655.

1. Start off at the lower calorie range. Counting calories is *not* necessary. For those who want to, however, 1,200 to 1,400 calories is a good place for most women to begin if they want to lose weight and are of average height (5' 4") and activity. It is easy to know where to start: just follow The Diet Solution Pyramid by eating the minimum number of servings suggested per day for each food group *and* choosing foods primarily from the four-star list provided by the Oregon Dairy Council. (Remember, you *can* have that occasional dessert, if you really want.) If you lose more than two pounds per week, add another serving of a four-star food from one of the groups. Likewise, do not eat fewer than the minimum number of servings recommended per day, even if you do not see immediate results. You will eventually. The minimum number of servings was calculated to give you just the right amounts of vitamins, minerals, carbohydrates, and protein that your body needs.

2. When you are ready to eat more (it won't happen at the same time for everyone, but you should be able to tell

when your body is ready), you can try going up to the mid-calorie range (for those who are counting, this is between 1,400 and 1,600 calories a day.) To do this, stick with eating the minimum number of servings, but add to your food choices by selecting from the three-star listings as well as the four. Monitor how you are doing. You can add or subtract the number of servings and change the nutrient categories accordingly. Your activity level should be increasing as well, so keep exercising.

3. When you have reached your desired weight, or even before, depending on your level of activity, your age, and your unique body, start eating in the maintenance range (between 1,600 and 1,800 calories a day). This means you will still be eating the minimum number of servings each day, but the range of foods to choose from can now include those in the two-star category. It is easy to adjust your choices if you find you need to. You may decide to choose two-star foods only occasionally, and instead eat more servings from the fruit, vegetable, and bread groups. You will still need to eat the minimum number of servings from each group. Don't cut out one serving of milk in order to eat more fruits, vegetables, and bread. Because most of the vegetables are so low in calories and fat, you should be able to eat more servings from this food group anyway. The more you exercise, the more liberal you can be in your choices.

This is very important: Eat the maximum calories you can while still losing weight. In other words, if you are losing 1½ to 2 pounds a week on 1,400 calories per day, don't drop to 1,200 calories. You will be more likely to stick with your diet and you will have more energy if you take this approach.

If you do not need to lose weight, but just want to have a healthier diet, choose foods from the four-star and three-star categories, keeping desserts and fatty foods to a minimum. Keep exercising.

Pregnant or nursing women, older adults, teenagers, children, athletes, and men each have different food needs. Most children, teenage girls, *active* women, and sedentary men need to eat more than the minimum but less than the maximum number of servings recommended for each food group. Active men, very active women, and teenage boys are usually best off when they consume the maximum number of servings recommended on the pyramid. Women who are pregnant or breast-feeding, teenagers, children, and young adults under the age of twenty-four need three servings per day from the milk group. Nursing or pregnant women should not diet. If you are pregnant or nursing, ask your doctor how many extra calories you need each day. Check with your doctor to know how much your child or teen should be eating.

As you analyze your own diet and begin to think of healthier ways to feed your family, determine which food groups you need to eat more of and which you need to eat less of. Most of us eat too few vegetables. There is not a law that says you can serve only one type of vegetable at dinner. Try small portions of a variety of vegetables. In many homes a scoop of peas or corn is the only vegetable eaten during the day. That makes up only one serving. On the other hand, when it comes to meat we often eat the maximum amount or more every day. Remember that one serving of meat is only two to three ounces in weight. If the recommended six servings of breads and cereals sounds like a lot, look at it this way: a small bowl of cereal and a piece of toast make two servings. Most of us have more than one ounce of cereal at a time, so breakfast is usually closer to three servings. A sandwich is two servings. A half-cup of pasta adds another serving. Now you are already up to six servings. If you want some crackers during the day as part of your snack (three or four counts as a serving), you should have the smaller bowl of cereal, or make your sandwich with only one slice of bread.

Following are breakfast, lunch, dinner, and snack ideas for the low-calorie plan. The low-calorie plan (1,200–1,400 calories per day) works best for women over thirty. If you are younger or do not need to lose very much weight (less than ten pounds), you can get by with eating more calories and exercising a bit more. You will learn what works best for *your* body as you fine-tune the Diet Solution to fit your needs. I encourage you to make up your own menus. Recipes for the starred items are included in chapter 5.

Breakfast

1 cup mixed fruit—kiwi, strawberries, and mandarin oranges (2 fruits)
½ cup plain yogurt (½ milk)—try flavoring the yogurt with a little vanilla or cinnamon
1 slice whole-wheat toast with a little butter or margarine (1 bread)

1 egg, fried, using vegetable spray (½ meat)
1 slice whole-wheat toast with a little butter or margarine (l bread)
½ grapefruit (1 fruit)

1 cup cooked whole-grain cereal (2 breads)
1 cup skim milk (1 milk)
6 ounces orange juice (1 fruit)

1 whole-grain bagel with a little butter or margarine (2 breads)
1 cup fruit smoothie* (1 fruit, 1 milk)

1 cup shredded wheat with small banana (2 breads, 1 fruit), or any cold cereal with ½ cup sliced fruit,
½ cup skim milk (½ milk)
1 slice toast with a little butter or margarine (1 bread)

2 fruit bran muffins* (2 breads, 1 fruit)
1 cup skim milk (1 milk)

½ toasted whole-wheat English muffin with 1 slice tomato and 1 thin
   slice low-fat cheese, broiled (I bread, ½ milk)
½ grapefruit (1 fruit)
½ cup skim milk (½ milk)

1 cup homemade granola* (2 breads, ½ meat, 1 fruit)
1 cup skim milk (1 milk)

2 eggs, scrambled, using one yolk and two whites (1 meat)
1 piece whole-wheat toast with 1 tbsp. jam (1 bread, ½ fruit)
½ cup strawberries (1 fruit)
1 cup skim milk (1 milk)

1 whole-wheat tortilla with 1 scrambled egg and 1 tbsp. salsa
   (1 bread, ½ meat)
6 ounces fruit juice (1 fruit)

1 2-egg omelet with mushrooms, onions, peppers, sprouts, tomatoes
   (1 meat, 1 vegetable)
½ whole-grain English muffin with a little butter or margarine (1
   bread)
1 orange (1 fruit)

Lunch

You can take many of these to work with you, or eat
equivalents if you are going out to lunch. Have with ice
water and a slice of lemon.

½ can tuna (1 meat)
1 cup chopped tomato and celery (1 vegetable)
1 cup lettuce and/or spinach (1 vegetable)
1 whole-wheat roll (1 bread)
1 cup plain nonfat yogurt (1 milk)

1 corn tortilla, cooked a few seconds on each side in pan sprayed
   with vegetable oil (1 bread)
Filling of ½ can vegetarian no-fat chili or other bean (1 meat)
Chopped lettuce and tomatoes (1 vegetable)
1½ ounces grated nonfat cheese (1 milk)

1 ½ cups white bean soup* (1 vegetable, 1 meat)
1 whole-wheat roll (1 bread)
1 cup lettuce and/or spinach with 1 tbsp. low-calorie dressing
    (1 vegetable)

½ whole-wheat pita (1 bread) filled with:
2 ounces chopped chicken mixed with 1 tsp. low-fat mayo (1 meat)
Chopped onion, tomato, and celery (1 vegetable)

2 slices whole-wheat bread (2 breads) topped and broiled with:
cucumber and tomato slices (1 vegetable)
1 ½ ounces low-fat cheese, sliced thin (1 milk)

½ whole-grain English muffin (1 bread) topped and broiled with:
2 ounces thin-sliced turkey ham (1 meat)
1 thin slice low-fat cheese (½ milk)
1 tomato, sliced (1 vegetable)

1 ½ cups minestrone soup* (1 meat, 1 vegetable)
1 whole-wheat roll with a little butter or margarine (1 bread)
1 cup lettuce and/or spinach with 1 tbsp. low-fat/low-calorie dressing
    (1 vegetable)

Egg-salad sandwich with 1 egg and 1 tsp. low-fat mayo (½ meat)
2 slices whole-grain bread (2 breads)
1 cup cooked green beans with a little butter or margarine (2 vegetables)

1 cup carrot-raisin salad* (1 vegetable, 1 fruit, ½ milk)
4 small, plain whole-grain crackers (1 bread)
1 cup vegetable soup* (1 vegetable)

Tuna salad with ½ can tuna, 1 tbsp. low-fat mayonnaise, and
    chopped cucumbers (1 meat, ½ vegetable)
2 slices whole-grain bread (2 breads)
1 cantaloupe section, approximately ¼ of the fruit (1 fruit)

Quesadillas* (2 bread, 1 milk, 1 vegetable)
1 hard-boiled egg (½ meat)
½ mango or papaya (1 fruit)

1 tomato, stuffed with 3 ounces canned salmon, mixed with 1 tbsp.
    low-fat mayo (1 vegetable, 1 meat)
½ whole-wheat roll (1 bread)

1 small baked potato (1 vegetable) topped with:
1 cup vegetarian low-fat chili or refried beans (½ meat)
1½ ounces low-fat cheese (1 milk)
1 cup lettuce/spinach salad with 1 tbsp. low-fat dressing
    (1 vegetable)

1 small baked potato (1 vegetable) topped with:
½ cup cooked broccoli (1 vegetable)
1½ ounces low-fat cheese (1 milk)
½ cup kiwi and strawberries (1 fruit)

1 cup whole-wheat pasta or regular pasta (2 breads)
½ cup homemade sauce* (½ vegetable)
1 cup cooked broccoli (2 vegetables)

3 ounces lean roast beef, turkey, or chicken (1 meat) on
2 slices rye or whole-wheat bread (2 breads)
2 tbsp. low-fat mayonnaise
1 cup lettuce with 1 chopped tomato, celery, sprouts
    (2 vegetables)

Dinner

Have these meals with water or milk, depending on the
number of milk servings you have already had for the day.

If you didn't have a leafy salad for lunch, have one for
dinner. Count the salad as one or two vegetables, depending on the veggies you add to the greens. In keeping with
the principle of eating meat sparingly, try not to have meat
for dinner if you had meat for lunch (this does not include

fish, which can be eaten more often because it is lower in fat, calories, and cholesterol than other meats). Choose a meat substitute instead. Some days try to have meat substitutes for both lunch and dinner. For example, have an omelet for lunch and a vegetable or bean soup for dinner. Check the number of servings you've had so far in the day.

Tuna pasta salad* (1 meat, 1 fruit, 2 breads)
1 cup cooked carrots or broccoli (2 vegetables)

Turkey casserole* with broccoli and brown rice (1 meat, 1 vegetable, 2 breads)
1 cup roasted green and red peppers (2 vegetables)

1 cup whole-grain spaghetti with homemade sauce (2 breads, 2 vegetables)
1 cup steamed green beans with oregano (2 vegetables)

1 small sweet potato with a little butter and ½ tsp. brown sugar, if desired (1 vegetable)
1 cup broccoli (2 vegetables)
3 ounces any type baked fish, with low-fat sauce (1 meat)
1 whole-wheat roll (1 bread)

Stuffed baked potato with: (1 vegetable)
1 ½ ounces cheese (1 milk)
½ cup broccoli or ½ cup vegetarian low-fat chili (1 vegetable or 1 meat)

Fish stew* (1 or 2 meats, 1 or 2 vegetables)
1 whole-grain roll (1 bread)
Lettuce and spinach salad with low-fat, low-calorie dressing (1 vegetable)

Oriental pork tenderloin with teriyaki or sweet and sour sauce, pineapple, and green peppers (1 meat, 1 fruit, 1 vegetable)
1 cup brown rice or mixed brown and white rice (2 breads)

Italian chicken* (1 meat, 1 vegetable)
1 small baked potato (1 vegetable)
1 cup lightly buttered green beans (1 vegetable)

Curried chicken* (1 meat)
½ or 1 cup wild rice (1 or 2 breads)
½ cup peas (1 vegetable)

Bagel pizza* (2 breads, 1 milk, 1 vegetable)
Lettuce and spinach salad with low-fat, low-calorie dressing (1 vegetable)

2 tortillas with ½ cup black beans and salsa (2 breads, 1 meat)
½ cup cooked corn, lightly buttered (1 vegetable)
1 orange (1 fruit)

2-egg omelet with vegetables (1 meat, 1 vegetable)
1 roasted potato (1 vegetable)

Fish Parmesan* (1 meat, 1 milk)
½ cup wild or brown rice (1 bread)
½ cup cooked carrots (1 vegetable)

Chicken dijon* (1 meat)
½ cup whole-wheat pasta with a little butter (1 bread)
½ cup cooked green beans (1 vegetable)

Bean and rice casserole* (1 meat, 1 bread)
Green salad with low-calorie, low-fat dressing (1 vegetable)
Cold vegetable plate with plain yogurt dip (1 or 2 vegetables, 1 milk)

Snacks

Snacks are optional, but you may eat one to three per day. Don't forget, however, that they contribute to your overall daily consumption from each food group.

Vegetable platter of carrots, snow peas, cauliflower, and broccoli
(1 or 2 vegetables). This can be served with nonfat plain yogurt for
a dip (½ milk).
Fruit, especially those with four stars (1 fruit)
1 cup plain, air-popped popcorn. If you buy the packaged microwave
kind, make sure there is no fat (3 cups plain=1 bread).
½ whole-grain English muffin (1 bread)
½ cup plain, low-fat yogurt with 3 or 4 whole-grain crackers (½ milk,
1 bread)

If you are following the mid-calorie plan, use fruits and
vegetables from all the categories in Pyramid Plus and try
three-starred items from the other food groups. When you
are eating at the maintenance level, choose from the two-
star range occasionally. Your menus can now include: a
wider selection of cuts of meat; more white potatoes; whole-
grain pancakes or waffles for any meal; pita bread; baked
corn tortilla chips with salsa for a snack or graham crackers.
Snacks can also include ⅓ cup nuts as well as frozen fruit-
juice bars. Instead of choosing some of the higher-calorie
foods, you may choose to eat more or larger servings of the
low-calorie foods. Monitor your progress and be aware of
the number of servings and serving sizes you eat each day.

4

HEALTH AND NUTRITION

"The fulness of the earth is yours, the beasts of the field and the fowls of the air, . . . and the herb, and the good things which come of the earth. . . . Yea, all things which come of the earth, in the season thereof, are made for the benefit and the use of man, both to please the eye and to gladden the heart; Yea, for food and for raiment, for taste and for smell, to strengthen the body and to enliven the soul."

—D&C 59:16–19

"The first principle that pertains to the intelligence God has bestowed upon us," Brigham Young said, "is to know how to preserve the present organization with which we are endowed. It is man's first duty to his existence, a knowledge of which would cause him to use all prudent efforts for the preservation of his life on the earth until his work here is completed."[22]

We have been given the fulness of the earth—a variety of foods divinely provided to supply all the nutrients our bodies need. It is our duty, according to Brigham Young, to understand this blessing and know how to use these foods to our benefit. In doing so, we can be healthy and strong and accomplish our purposes in this life.

Your health is compromised if you are overweight. The National Institute of Health reports that "if you are a woman and your waist measures more than 35 inches, or if you are a man and your waist measures more than 40 inches, you are more likely to develop heart disease, high blood pressure, diabetes, and certain cancers. . . . Overweight people are twice as likely to develop type 2 diabetes (non-insulin-dependent) as people who are not overweight."[23] Studies show that even losing ten or twenty pounds can improve your health. Staying healthy is more than just losing weight or eating right; you also need to exercise and have regular physical checkups.

After the release of the American Cancer Society's study on obesity in *The New England Journal of Medicine* in October 1999, JoAnn Manson, a Harvard University endocrinologist and preventive-health specialist, said: "The evidence is now compelling and irrefutable. Obesity is probably the second-leading preventable cause of death in the United States after cigarette smoking, so it is a very serious problem."[24] The lead author of the study, Eugenia Calle, said: "The message is we're too fat and it's killing us. We need to come up with ways as a society to eat less and exercise more."[25] Here is what Brigham Young had to say on the subject: " . . . eat less, and we shall be a great deal wiser, healthier, and wealthier people than by taking the course we now do."[26] And on another occasion he told the Saints: "Now I do not mean fasting, but eating moderately; . . . commence to adopt this rule, you will find that you begin to get better. . . . We do not expect all to be free from sickness. . . . But we can amend our ways, and amend our life by being prudent."[27] By moderating your diet, as Brigham Young suggested, you may be able to win the fight against two of America's leading killers: heart disease and cancer.

HEART DISEASE

The amount of cholesterol in the blood is affected by the amount of saturated fat and cholesterol in the foods you eat. Because the body produces its own cholesterol, mostly in the liver, heredity also affects your cholesterol level. Cholesterol is measured in milligrams per deciliter of blood (mg/dL). High cholesterol levels (higher than 200 mg/dL) can lead to atherosclerosis, or narrowing of the arteries, which can cause a heart attack or stroke. (Some experts say anything higher than 150 mg/dL is risky.)

In talking about cholesterol, you have probably heard the terms HDL, or "good" cholesterol, and LDL, or "bad" cholesterol. HDL cholesterol moves quickly through the bloodstream, while LDL cholesterol is less dense and moves more slowly, therefore contributing to plaque buildup in the arteries. Think of HDL as a marble that speeds through the bloodstream and LDL as a marshmallow that sort of slogs its way through.

Most saturated fat comes from animal products, such as meat, butter, cream, whole milk, cheese, and ice cream. Some saturated fat comes from plants, such as coconut oil, cocoa butter, and palm oil. Cholesterol is found only in animal products—eggs, meat, poultry, fish, and dairy. Vegetables, nuts, grains, and cereals do not contain cholesterol. By substituting unsaturated fats for saturated fats, you can lower cholesterol levels and reduce your risk of heart disease. Unsaturated fats can be found in olive oil, safflower, corn, soybean, and canola oils. Butter has saturated fat, margarine does not. However, I much prefer the taste of butter, so I put butter on my food, but in such small amounts that it doesn't matter. When I bake, it depends on the recipe. Some baked goods really need butter, so I use it. When it does not make a difference, I use margarine.

Breaking Down Cholesterol

Form of Cholesterol	Low Risk	Moderate Risk	High Risk
Total cholesterol	Less than 200 mg/dL	200–239 mg/dL	240 mg/dL and over
LDL cholesterol	Less than 130 mg/dL	130–159 mg/dL	160 mg/dL and over
HDL cholesterol	35 mg/dL and over	Less than 35 mg/dL	Less than 35 mg/dL

Source: Lori A. Smolin and Mary B. Grosvenor, *Nutrition: Science & Applications* (Orlando, Florida: Harcourt, Inc., 2000), p. 143.

Know Your Blood Pressure

Hypertension, or high blood pressure, causes your heart to work harder to pump blood and oxygen through your body. This increases your risk of heart attack, stroke, kidney failure, and atherosclerosis. You should have your blood pressure checked regularly. For some people, one way to lower high blood pressure is to eat less salt. One teaspoon of salt contains about 2,000 mg of sodium, which is close to the upper limit recommended by many health authorities: 2,400 mg of sodium per day. I have stopped putting salt on the table. My cupboard is lined with pretty, but unused, saltshakers. (It's important to recognize that most of our salt does not come from what we add at the table. Most of our salt comes from processed and prepared foods.) I still cook with salt, but I have found I can reduce the amount called for in recipes and not tell any difference in the outcome. Buy low-salt products whenever possible and rinse canned tuna and vegetables to remove much of the salt. Many packaged foods are high in salt, especially soups. Cook from scratch as much as you can. And be aware that restaurants often use more salt than you would at home. Try seasoning with herbs instead of salt. I have included in appendix L a list of herbs and spices that can liven up the taste of various foods.

What Do the Numbers Mean?

The systolic number is always stated first and the diastolic number is listed second. For example: 122/76 (122 over 76); systolic = 122, diastolic = 76.

• The higher (systolic) number represents the pressure while the heart is beating.

• The lower (diastolic) number represents the pressure when the heart is resting between beats.

Blood pressure lower than 140 over 90 is considered normal for adults. A systolic pressure of 130 to 139 or a diastolic pressure of 85 to 89 should be carefully watched. A reading equal to or higher than 140 over 90 is considered elevated or high.

CANCER

The National Cancer Institute estimates that about one-third of all cancer deaths may be related to the foods we eat. The Institute's studies show that diets high in fiber can reduce colon and rectum cancer.[28] Whole-grain breads and cereals, vegetables, fruits, and beans are all good sources of fiber. Eat the foods, not supplements. Fiber in your diet not only makes you feel full, it also speeds up the passage of food through the intestines so that your tissues are not exposed to cancer-causing agents in food for long periods of time. Do not overload on fiber—more than 35 grams per day is too much. Drink more water as you eat more fiber. In appendix J is a chart showing the fiber content of several foods.

High-fat diets have been shown to contribute to breast, colon, uterine, and prostate cancer. Eating foods rich in vitamin A, vitamin C, and beta-carotene may help reduce the risk of certain cancers. Choose yellow-orange vegetables such as carrots, winter squash, sweet potatoes, and pumpkin for vitamin A and beta-carotene. Yellow-orange fruits such as peaches, cantaloupes, and mangoes are also high in vitamin A.

Vitamin E is an antioxidant, which means it protects the body against cell and tissue damage caused when the cells burn oxygen. Almonds are especially high in vitamin E. You can also get the vitamin from other nuts, peanut butter, seeds, green leafy vegetables, and whole-grain products. Vitamin C and beta-carotene are also antioxidants.

Vitamin C is found in dark-green leafy vegetables such as spinach, kale, and watercress and in broccoli, asparagus, and tomatoes. Fruits that supply vitamin C include oranges, lemons, grapefruit, cantaloupe, and berries. Cabbage family vegetables such as cabbage, broccoli, cauliflower, brussels sprouts, radishes, turnips, mustard greens, kale, kohlrabi, and watercress have been found to help protect against colon cancer and are also good sources of fiber.[29] *The Journal of the American Medical Association* published an interesting study on these groups of fruits and vegetables in October 1999. The study, conducted by the Harvard School of Public Health, concluded that eating more fruits and vegetables lowers the risk of stroke. Vegetables in the cabbage family were especially beneficial.[30] I happen to love brussels sprouts, but strangely, a lot of people don't, including my husband. Because I've been telling him how good they are at fighting colon cancer, he has been willing to eat a few. Of course, there are many other vegetables in this category from which to choose.

OSTEOPOROSIS

Osteoporosis, though usually not life-threatening, is also preventable through proper diet and exercise. Osteoporosis is the gradual loss of bone mass, often caused by lack of calcium. To prevent it, eat foods rich in calcium, buy calcium-fortified products, take calcium supplements if necessary, and exercise to promote healthy bone tissue. Even sunlight can help. Vitamin D aids in calcium absorption and is produced by your skin when you are in the sun.

The out-of-doors can be very therapeutic, especially in the winter when you may suffer from sensory deprivation and, therefore, want to eat more. Wearing a good sunscreen is a must, both to prevent skin cancer and to combat the effects of aging. There is no sense in sabotaging your efforts by having leathery, old-looking skin. Sunscreen will keep the skin from producing vitamin D, so put sunscreen on after twenty minutes of sun exposure, or just put it on your face to start. The National Academy of Sciences recommends that women age nineteen to fifty-one have 1,000 mg of calcium per day. Teenagers and nursing mothers need about 1,300 mg. You'll need 1,200 mg if you are entering menopause. The best sources for calcium are dairy products, tofu, green leafy vegetables, salmon, sardines with bones, and calcium-fortified orange juice.

NUTRITION FACTS

The Nutrition Facts label on most prepared foods is an invaluable resource for people who want to incorporate healthier food choices into their diets. Before 1994 the food industry was not required to provide nutritional information to the consumer. Therefore, a lot of what you chose to buy was based on guesswork and advertising claims. But now labeling is mandatory, and you should make it a habit to read the nutrition label on everything you buy.

Deciphering the Label

Following is a breakdown of each of the features on the Nutrition Facts label:

• *Serving Size*—The serving size approximates how much most people eat. The nutritional information on labels is based on the serving amount. If you eat more or less than the serving size shown on the label, the amount of calories, fat, and nutrients you take in goes up or down.

• *Calories*—This shows how many calories are in a single serving and how many of the calories come from fat.

• *% Daily Values*—The term "% Daily Value" refers to the percentage (per serving) of the recommended daily intake of important vitamins and minerals, carbohydrates, dietary fiber, and protein, as well as fat, cholesterol, and sodium that is in a food, based on a 2,000-calorie diet. It is important to remember that some Daily Values are presented as minimums while others are maximums. Calcium is one example of a minimum. If a food contains only 20 percent of the daily value of calcium (based on a 2,000-calorie diet), you would need to eat *at least* five servings of that food to get enough calcium for the day. Fat, on the other hand, is a maximum. If one serving of a particular food contains 20 percent of the recommended daily value of fat, it means five servings of that food have all the fat you *should* eat in one day based on a 2,000-calorie diet. (But you should probably eat less than that if you're trying to lose weight.) Your daily values will change from those listed on the label if your calorie intake is higher or lower than two thousand.

• *Dietary Components*—All Nutrition Facts labels contain lists of nutrients and other dietary components so that you can make informed choices about what you are eating. In most cases your goal is to get 100 percent of the daily value for the vitamins—particularly A and C—and the minerals—calcium, iron, and so on. The fat component on the label is broken down to show how much of the total fat is saturated. Choose more often foods that are lower in saturated fat. The carbohydrates component is also divided into two important features: fiber and sugar. Look for foods higher in fiber and lower in sugar.

• *Ingredients*—This section of the label lists by weight the ingredients in the food. Be especially aware of the first three ingredients listed. This will tell you a lot about what your family is eating.

To help you learn how to read and interpret food labels, let's compare the labels from two boxes of cereal. If you primarily eat cold cereal for breakfast (using skim milk or 1 percent milk with it), you should vary your cereals and look for ones higher in fiber and vitamins and lower in fat and sugar. On the following page are the labels from a box of Trix and a box of Cheerios. Cheerios is the healthier choice of these two cereals. It has more protein, more vitamins, more fiber, and far less sugar. (A cereal with at least three grams of fiber is best.) Now look at the first three items in each ingredients list. Trix lists corn meal (not much fiber), and then two sugar sources, regular sugar and corn syrup. Cheerios lists whole grain oats (plenty of fiber), modified corn starch, and then wheat starch (even more fiber). Sugar is fourth on the ingredients list. I am not suggesting that your child should never eat Trix or similar cereals. Trix is fortified with many vitamins and is low in fat. I let my son have it once in a while, and then I supplement it with whole-wheat toast and put bananas on the cereal.

When I was a child, my mother did not give us cold cereal for breakfast during the school year. If we had cereal, it was hot cereal. I felt sorry for my friends whose mothers fed them cold cereal—I didn't think they were being fed properly. But as you can see from looking at the labels, plain Cheerios, which has been around for a long time, is one of the healthiest cold cereals you can feed your family. It has 110 calories, 3 grams of fiber, 1 gram of sugar, and is made from whole-grain oats, which includes the oat bran. Some "adult" cold cereals, particularly the granola kind, that are promoted as healthy have high amounts of fat and sugar. One granola label I read showed that the cereal contained 17 grams of sugar, even more than Trix.

Because of the Nutrition Facts label, we now have much more control over our own health. Other information we need is available in many forms. Hospitals have wellness and nutrition clinics. Newspapers and magazines carry

Trix

Nutrition Facts

Serving Size 1 cup (30g)
Servings Per Container 16

Amount Per Serving		Trix	with 1/2 cup skim milk
Calories		120	160
Calories from Fat		15	15
		% Daily Value **	
Total Fat 1.5g*		**3%**	**3%**
Saturated Fat 0g		**0%**	**3%**
Polyunsaturated Fat 0g			
Monounsaturated Fat 0.5g			
Cholesterol 0mg		**0%**	**1%**
Sodium 200mg		**8%**	**11%**
Total Carbohydrate 26g		**9%**	**11%**
Dietary Fiber 1g		**4%**	**4%**
Sugars 13g			
Other Carbohydrate 12g			
Protein 1g			
Vitamin A		10%	15%
Vitamin C		10%	10%
Calcium		2%	15%
Iron		25%	25%
Vitamin D		10%	25%
Thiamin		25%	30%
Riboflavin		25%	35%
Niacin		25%	25%
Vitamin B6		25%	25%
Folic Acid		25%	25%
Vitamin B12		25%	35%
Zinc		25%	30%

*Amount in Cereal. A serving of cereal plus skim milk provides 2g fat (0.5g saturated fat), less than 5mg cholesterol, 260mg sodium, 32g total carbohydrate (19g sugars) and 5g protein.

**Percent Daily Values are based on a 2,000 calorie diet. Your daily values may be higher or lower depending on your calorie needs:

	Calories	2,000	2,500
Total Fat	Less than	65g	80g
Sat Fat	Less than	20g	25g
Cholesterol	Less than	300mg	300mg
Sodium	Less than	2,400mg	2,400mg
Total Carbohydrate		300g	375g
Dietary Fiber		25g	30g

INGREDIENTS: CORN MEAL, SUGAR, CORN SYRUP, PARTIALLY HYDROGENATED SOYBEAN AND/OR COTTONSEED OIL, MODIFIED CORN STARCH, WHEAT STARCH, SALT, GUAR GUM, GUM ARABIC, HIGH FRUCTOSE CORN SYRUP, DICALCIUM PHOSPHATE, CALCIUM CARBONATE, TRISODIUM PHOSPHATE, RED 40, YELLOW 6, BLUE 1 AND OTHER COLOR ADDED, BAKING SODA, NATURAL AND ARTIFICIAL FLAVOR, MALIC ACID, CITRIC ACID.

Cheerios

Nutrition Facts

Serving Size 1 cup (30g)
Servings Per Container About 14

Amount Per Serving		Cheerios	with 1/2 cup skim milk
Calories		110	150
Calories from Fat		15	20
		% Daily Value **	
Total Fat 2g*		**3%**	**3%**
Saturated Fat 0g		**0%**	**3%**
Polyunsaturated Fat 0.5g			
Monounsaturated Fat 0.5g			
Cholesterol 0mg		**0%**	**1%**
Sodium 280mg		**12%**	**15%**
Potassium 95mg		**3%**	**9%**
Total Carbohydrate 22g		**7%**	**9%**
Dietary Fiber 3g		**11%**	**11%**
Soluble Fiber 1g			
Sugars 1g			
Other Carbohydrate 18g			
Protein 3g			
Vitamin A		10%	15%
Vitamin C		10%	10%
Calcium		4%	20%
Iron		45%	45%
Vitamin D		10%	25%
Thiamin		25%	30%
Riboflavin		25%	35%
Niacin		25%	25%
Vitamin B6		25%	25%
Folic Acid		50%	50%
Vitamin B12		25%	35%
Phosphorus		10%	25%
Magnesium		8%	10%
Zinc		25%	30%
Copper		2%	2%

*Amount in Cereal. A serving of cereal plus skim milk provides 2g total fat (0.5g saturated fat, 1g monounsaturated fat), less than 5mg cholesterol, 350mg sodium, 300mg potassium, 28g total carbohydrate (7g sugars) and 7g protein.

**Percent Daily Values are based on a 2,000 calorie diet. Your daily values may be higher or lower depending on your calorie needs:

	Calories	2,000	2,500
Total Fat	Less than	65g	80g
Sat Fat	Less than	20g	25g
Cholesterol	Less than	300mg	300mg
Sodium	Less than	2,400mg	2,400mg
Potassium		3,500mg	3,500mg
Total Carbohydrate		300g	375g
Dietary Fiber		25g	30g

INGREDIENTS: WHOLE GRAIN OATS (INCLUDES THE OAT BRAN), MODIFIED CORN STARCH, WHEAT STARCH, SUGAR, SALT, OAT FIBER, TRISODIUM PHOSPHATE, CALCIUM CARBONATE, VITAMIN E (MIXED TOCOPHEROLS) ADDED TO PRESERVE FRESHNESS.

more articles about health. Web sites devoted to health topics proliferate on the Internet. I have included a list of some reliable Web sites in appendix A.

More than half of Americans are now overweight, according to the *Journal of the American Medical Association.* "The time has come to develop a national comprehensive obesity prevention strategy that incorporates educational, behavioral, and environmental components analogous to those already in place for tobacco use," the journal reported.[31] In other words, health experts believe our way of eating could be as dangerous to our health as cigarette smoking. No wonder the Word of Wisdom includes dietary guidelines as well as cautions against smoking and drinking.

Brigham Young said: "By and by, according to the Scriptures, the days of a man shall be like the days of a tree. But in those days people will not eat and drink as they do now; if they do their days will not be like a tree, unless it be a very short-lived tree." He went on to say, "The people have laid the foundation of short life through their diet." And, "As we . . . have lived more richly, indulging in sweet cake, plum pudding, roast beef and so on, we have had more or less disease among us." "Go into their houses and you will find beef, pork, apple pie, custard pie, pumpkin pie, mince pie, and every luxury, and they live so as to shorten their days and the days of their children." Then, in reference to the health guidelines in the Word of Wisdom, Brigham Young continued, " . . . but let the people observe them and they lay the foundation for longevity."[32]

Brigham Young was concerned, I think, with *overindulgence* in these rich foods.

5

MEAL PLANNING AND RECIPES

"The Americans, as a nation, are killing themselves with their vices and high living. As much as a man ought to eat in half an hour they swallow in three minutes, gulping down their food. . . . Dispense with your multitudinous dishes, and depend upon it, you will do much towards preserving your families from sickness, disease and death."

—Brigham Young

The Word of Wisdom provides the blueprint for a healthy life. Together with the Food Guide Pyramid and the Nutrition Facts label, you can plan a diet that contains the essential nutrients for good health and helps you lose weight, if that is part of your goal.

Your diet needs to have *adequate vitamins and minerals,* which come from eating a *variety* of foods from the food groups. Ask your doctor if you should also be taking a vitamin and mineral supplement. As you are planning your meals, remember to eat enough protein to preserve muscle tissue and repair body tissue. The average woman twenty-five years of age and older needs 50 grams of protein each day. For men the amount is 63 grams. If you are eating two to three servings from the meat group daily, you should be

56

fine. (Remember, the protein you need does not have to come primarily from meat.) You will also need at least 100 grams of carbohydrates per day just to keep up your energy and prevent fluid imbalances. Men need much more. The six to eleven servings from the bread group on the Food Guide Pyramid will do it. A daily fiber intake of 20 to 35 grams is recommended for proper bowel function. Limit your fat and cholesterol. Fewer than 30 percent of calories should come from fat per day. If you are trying to lose weight, you can trim this much lower. A good figure to go by is 30 *grams* of fat per day if you're eating in the lower-calorie plan (1,200–1,400 calories) and 35 grams of fat per day on the medium-calorie plan (1,400–1,600 calories). Most of the fat should be unsaturated. Cholesterol should be less than 300 mg daily, according to government experts. Other health experts suggest less. (A small hamburger has 100 mg of cholesterol and an egg contains about 215 mg.)[33]

Making healthier food choices becomes easier when we know what nutrients our bodies should have and what foods supply them. I have changed the way I grocery shop so that I am more aware of what I am buying. I also go to the grocery store once a month or even less frequently, except to pick up fresh produce. I can remember what it was like dragging little children to the grocery store once a week for a big shop. It was exhausting for all of us. Picking up produce just once a week, however, is easy. It has made a big difference in my food budget, and we are all eating better foods. I buy meats and other foods in large quantities and I shop case lot sales. I divide the meats up and repackage them in freezer bags. Having lived in an apartment in New York City, I recognize that shopping once a month may not be practical. There usually is not enough room to store the food, but what is in the cupboards and in the refrigerator can still be improved upon. The same goes for families whose budgets do not allow for a monthly shop.

SHOPPING FOR FOOD

Here are some suggestions for your next excursion to the grocery store:

• Significantly cut down on your meat purchases. This alone will reduce your food bill. The meats you buy should be lean cuts. Often the meat department will trim the remaining visible fat for you. You can also ask the butcher's advice for the leanest cuts of meat. These would include pork tenderloin, round tip roast, and sirloin. Buy more fish than you are accustomed to. Have cans of tuna, salmon, and clams on hand. Add them to pasta or beans for a quick meal. The white meat of poultry is lower in fat. Buy skinned chicken breast, or skin the chicken before you cook it. Cook a whole bird on a rack to keep it out of the drippings.

• Look for low-fat dairy products, such as skim or one-percent milk, low-fat or nonfat yogurt, and low-fat cheeses.

• Buy cooking oils that are unsaturated or monounsaturated, such as canola oil, corn oil, olive oil, and soybean oil.

• Select breads, bagels, and English muffins made from whole-wheat, rye, bran, or corn flour or corn meal. Read the Nutrition Facts label on the bread. I was surprised to learn that a brown bread I was regularly buying had only one gram of fiber, the same amount as in white bread. Even if the bread says "multigrain," check the label. Whole wheat or whole grain means the food contains a bran layer, which is the outer coating of the grain and is high in fiber.

• Buy whole-wheat flour, but keep it in the refrigerator or freezer, because its shelf life is shorter than white flour. You can also try whole-wheat pancake mixes. Try whole-grain or bran cereals, whole-wheat pasta, brown rice, and bulgur wheat. I have included a good bulgur wheat recipe. You do not need to switch entirely to whole grains. And definitely do not try to do so all at once—your body needs time to get used to digesting whole grains. Products made with white flour are not "bad." Because they are fortified they are still nutritious, but they do lack the fiber of whole-grain products. Try mixing brown and white rice, or whole-grain and regular pasta. Do not be fooled by colored pastas. Vegetable extracts are used to add color, but that is about all that is added. It is still regular pasta.

• Buy dry peas and beans, such as split peas, black-eyed peas, chickpeas, kidney beans, navy beans, and lentils. They are very inexpensive. You do not have to soak split peas or lentils. I have included recipes for dry peas and beans later in the book. If you buy canned beans, rinse the beans to remove the salt. Try vegetarian refried beans, chili, and baked beans. Use them as toppings on potatoes if you do not want to eat them plain. As little as one-half cup of beans is a good addition to your protein for the day. Taco shells and tortillas, especially the whole-wheat kind, are good sources of complex carbohydrates. Avoid pre-made taco shells when you can—they are deep fat fried. Buy them uncooked and fry your own by spraying a pan with a little vegetable spray and cooking on both sides for two minutes or less, then folding.

• Buy plenty of fresh fruit and vegetables. Did you know romaine lettuce has six times the vitamin C and eight times the beta-carotene as iceberg lettuce? Iceberg lettuce is not bad. But knowing this should help you to eat a variety of produce.

• Choose fresh produce, especially when the foods are in season. Any time the fruit or vegetable is processed, some of the nutrients are lost. If you keep the fresh produce in your refrigerator for a week or two, it will lose nutrients too. The best solution is to grow as much as you can and eat it immediately or process it immediately. Canned and dried fruit are good too, but they contain more sugar. Peaches in light syrup have two teaspoons of added sugar per half-cup serving; heavy syrup has four teaspoons of added sugar. Look for fruits packed in their own juices. Frozen berries are good to have on hand and they often are prepared without sugar. If you like canned vegetables, buy the no-salt or low-salt kind; all others can be rinsed. To get used to more variety, buy some vegetables you would not ordinarily choose.

PREPARING FOOD

When it comes time to prepare the foods, you again have choices that will result in healthier meals.

• Serve vegetables raw. You do not always have to serve cooked vegetables. Try carrots, broccoli, cauliflower, and snow peas.

• Steam your vegetables—you don't lose as many nutrients this way. When you do cook them in water, you may want to keep the lid on the pan so fewer nutrients escape with the steam. (After cooking vegetables, use the liquid in other dishes, as some of the vitamins will have dissolved in the water. You can also use leftover water for your plants.) The shorter the cooking time, the more nutrients you will preserve. High heat also destroys vitamins.

• Bake, steam, boil, microwave, or broil food instead of frying it. A fried pork chop has 16 grams of fat, while a lean piece of roast pork has half that amount. A three-ounce piece of fried chicken has 12 grams of fat, compared to a piece of baked chicken with 8 fat grams.

• Trim off the fat from meats, and skin poultry and fish.

• Skim fat from soups and gravies. After the soups or gravies are refrigerated it is even easier to take most of the fat out.

• Cook with skim milk.

• Use low-fat, low-calorie mayonnaise and salad dressings.

• Buy a vegetable brush and clean your fruits and vegetables thoroughly instead of peeling most of them. The skins of fruits and vegetables are loaded with fiber.

• Use low-fat yogurt instead of sour cream.

• Sauté or stir-fry; you will find that you can use a lot less fat when you do. Try using half as much oil as usual.

• Use one whole egg and one egg white in recipes—instead of two whole eggs—to cut cholesterol.

• Try whole-wheat pancakes, even for dinner, and top with applesauce or fresh berries instead of syrup.

• Make homemade soups and freeze enough for meals later. The soups do not have to be watery gruel. I have included in the recipe section a way to thicken soups without using a lot of fat.

• Use ⅓ less oil than the recipe calls for when baking. Experiment to see what works best for you.

For many busy women, all this may sound like too much time and work, especially if feeding a family. The temptation is to get take-out or buy packaged foods. I have found a couple of ways around this: the Crock-Pot and the pressure cooker. A Crock-Pot will cook your meal all day and be ready for you by dinnertime. If you have not used your Crock-Pot for years, food safety experts advise checking it. Slow cooking can provide an environment in which harmful bacteria thrive. You do not have to worry about new Crock-Pots. Test your old Crock-Pot by putting water in it and setting it on low. Before two hours is up the temperature must have reached 165° F. Check it with a thermometer. If it has not reached 165° F., set it on high until it does. Then turn it back to low. It must maintain 140° F. at this setting. This means you can use it, but you would have to use the high setting and be home to turn it down.

Pressure cookers are no longer scary. They come in several sizes and are easy and safe to use. You can have a healthy meal—preserving many of the nutrients that are lost in longer cooking methods—in the time it takes to go out and buy something. Pressure cookers can literally cook a dinner in minutes. At 4:00 P.M. do you know what you are fixing for dinner? Even if you are using conventional cooking methods a healthy meal can take a minimum amount of time to prepare. Have the basics on hand. Thin cuts of meat and fish cook quickly. Bagged vegetables and salads are quick and easy. Always wash the produce thoroughly, even if the package says it's "pre-washed." Food poisoning has been known to happen even with "pre-washed" produce, because "pre-washed" and "triple washed" sometimes mean washing over and over in the same dirty water. With a selection of canned beans, such as cannellini, garbanzo, black, kidney, and navy; some lettuce or spinach; a variety of pastas; and corn, peas, or tomatoes, you can put together several nutritious complete-protein meals in a hurry. Add a little low-fat or fat-free dressing, if you like. There are a lot of tasty dressings on the market now. You do not have to confine yourself to ranch or Italian.

Home economists from Utah State University have cited studies that show families eat the same ten main-food dishes 80 percent of the time. Take a look at your typical meals. Make a list of all the main dishes frequently eaten and add foods from the food pyramid that would make the dishes healthier. Look at how you usually prepare those meals and see if there are ways to cut back on the fat and salt. See how many of the dishes could be prepared without meat or with a protein substitute. If you have a family, it might be fun and helpful to do this as a family project and get everyone involved. Talk about some new menus you could try. Look over vegetarian cookbooks in your library or bookstore and find one that has recipes you think you or your family would eat on occasion. (I am not advocating, however, that you become a vegetarian.) The Seventh-Day Adventist Church, whose members are vegetarians, has many ideas for cooking without meat while still getting the necessary protein. You can contact your local Seventh-Day Adventist Church for information on their products. Some of the recipes that follow are from the nutrition department of Loma Linda University, a Seventh-Day Adventist school. Other recipes, with meat and without, come from the National Cancer Institute, the National Institute of Health, the Produce for Better Health Institute, and the Salt Lake City Extension office of Utah State University. (All states have extension offices. Check your local extension office for more recipes.) Most of the recipes include nutritional information. Some of the older recipes I've included do not; nonetheless, they are still low in fat and healthy.

RECIPES

Pineapple Sweet Potatoes

$\frac{1}{2}$ tablespoon margarine
8-ounce can crushed
   pineapple in natural juice
2 cups fresh sweet potatoes,
   cooked and sliced

$\frac{1}{4}$ teaspoon cinnamon
$\frac{1}{8}$ teaspoon salt

Heat margarine in a large frying pan. Add sweet potato slices and pineapple. Sprinkle with cinnamon and salt. Simmer uncovered until most of the juice has cooked away. This may take 10 to 15 minutes. Turn potato slices a few times to coat them with the pineapple juice, then serve. Makes 4 servings.

Source: United States Department of Agriculture.

Zucchini Tuna Canoes

2 small zucchini
   (each about 6 inches long)
6.5-ounce can tuna,
   drained, flaked

3 tablespoons salad dressing
$\frac{1}{2}$ teaspoon dill weed
$\frac{1}{4}$ teaspoon onion powder
16 (1-inch) carrot sticks

Cut zucchini in half lengthwise. Cut a thin slice from the bottom of each half so they sit upright. Scoop out center of each half, leaving about $\frac{1}{4}$-inch shell; set aside. Combine tuna, salad dressing, dill weed, and onion powder. Spoon tuna mixture into zucchini halves. Cover; refrigerate and serve. Cut each "canoe" in half; insert carrot stick on each side of tuna mixture to form paddles, and serve. Makes 8 servings.

Source: Utah State University Extension, Salt Lake County.

Herbed Vegetable Combo

These steamed vegetables with herb seasonings add color and flavor to a meal without adding fat or salt.

2 tablespoons water
1 cup zucchini squash,
   thinly sliced
$1\frac{1}{4}$ cups yellow squash,
   thinly sliced
$\frac{1}{2}$ cup green pepper,
   cut into 2-inch strips

$\frac{1}{4}$ cup celery, cut into
   2-inch strips
$\frac{1}{4}$ cup onion, chopped
$\frac{1}{2}$ teaspoon caraway seed
$\frac{1}{8}$ teaspoon garlic powder
1 medium tomato,
   cut into 8 wedges

Heat water in large frying pan. Add squash, green pepper, celery, and onion. Cover and cook over moderate heat until vegetables are tender-crisp—about 4 minutes. Sprinkle seasonings over vegetables. Top with tomato wedges. Cover and cook over low heat until tomato wedges are just heated—about 2 minutes. Makes 4 $\frac{3}{4}$-cup servings

Each serving provides: 25 calories, trace total fat, trace saturated fatty acids, 0 mg cholesterol, 10 mg sodium.

Source: United States Department of Agriculture.

Baked Apples

4 medium cooking apples
4 tablespoons raisins
¾ cup water
½ teaspoon cinnamon

Preheat oven to 350°F. Remove cores from apples, leaving ½ inch of the core at bottom of the apple. Peel top one-third of apple. Arrange apples in baking pan. Put 1 tablespoon of raisins in the center of each apple. Pour water over apples. Sprinkle cinnamon over apples. Bake 45 to 60 minutes or until tender. Spoon liquid from pan over apples one or two times during baking. Makes 4 servings; 1 apple each.

Each serving provides: 150 calories, 1 g total fat, 0 mg cholesterol, 0 mg sodium.

Source: United States Department of Agriculture

Carrot Raisin Salad*

2 cups shredded carrots
½ cup raisins
2 tablespoons fat-free mayonnaise
¼ cup plain, nonfat yogurt
2 tablespoons lemon juice

Shred carrots and combine with other ingredients; chill. Makes 6 servings.

Each serving provides: 74 calories, 21% DV total fat, 2 mg cholesterol, 56 mg sodium, 74% DV carbohydrate, 5% DV protein, 33 mg. calcium, 0.5 mg iron.

Source: University of Utah Nutrition Clinic.

Pasta Salad

³/₄ cup elbow macaroni,   2 tablespoons onion, chopped
  uncooked   ¹/₄ cup low-fat Italian dressing
10-ounce package frozen
  mixed vegetables
¹/₃ medium green pepper, chopped

Cook macaroni and frozen vegetables according to package directions. Leave out the salt. Drain. Add the green pepper, onion, and low-fat Italian dressing. Mix all ingredients. Chill well. Makes 4 one-cup servings.

Each serving provides: 135 calories, 2 g total fat, 0 mg cholesterol, 145 mg sodium.

Source: United States Department of Agriculture.

Crunchy Pea Salad

1¹/₂ cups USA split peas, rinsed   8-ounce can water chestnuts,
3 cups water   diced
1¹/₂ cups instant rice, cooked   3 bunches green onions,
¹/₂ cup chopped celery   chopped

Dressing:
1 cup cholesterol-free mayonnaise   1 tablespoon horseradish
¹/₂ cup chili sauce   (optional)
Few drops Tabasco sauce   ¹/₄ cup sweet red pepper sauce
                                        (optional)

Cook the split peas in boiling water for 25 to 30 minutes. Peas should be tender, not mushy. Drain, rinse, and chill. Chill cooked rice. Combine the peas and rice with the water chestnuts, green onions, and celery. Serve with dressing.

For dressing combine mayonnaise, chili sauce, Tabasco sauce, horseradish, and pepper sauce. Serves 12.

Each serving provides: 256 calories, 9 g total fat, 0 mg cholesterol, 206 mg sodium, 38 g carbohydrate, 1 g dietary fiber, 6 g protein.

Source: USA Dry Pea and Lentil Council, Moscow, Idaho.

Lentil Confetti Salad

1 cup USA lentils, rinsed
3 cups water
1 cup rice, cooked and warm
$\frac{1}{2}$ cup light Italian dressing
1 large tomato, seeded and diced
1 tablespoon parsley, chopped

$\frac{1}{2}$ cup onion, chopped
$\frac{1}{2}$ cup celery, chopped
$\frac{1}{4}$ cup pimento-stuffed olives, sliced
$\frac{1}{4}$ cup sweet green pepper, diced

Garnish :
cucumbers and red onion rings, sliced

In a saucepan, pour water over lentils, bring to a boil, and simmer 20 minutes or until lentils are tender. Combine drained lentils with rice and all vegetables. Toss lightly with dressing. Place on a ring of cucumbers and garnish with red onion rings. Serves 8.

Each serving provides: 231 calories, 8 g total fat, 0 mg cholesterol, 324 mg sodium, 22 g carbohydrate, 2.5 g dietary fiber, 3.5 g protein.

Source: USA Dry Pea and Lentil Council, Moscow, Idaho.

Diced Chik and Black Bean Salad

2 tablespoons olive oil
2 tablespoons fresh cilantro, chopped
2 tablespoons fresh lime juice
1 teaspoon sugar
1 clove garlic, minced
$\frac{1}{2}$ teaspoon chili powder
$\frac{1}{3}$ cup sliced green onions

13-ounce can low-fat Worthington Diced Chik, well drained
1 15-ounce can black beans, rinsed and drained
1 15-ounce can whole kernel corn, drained
1 red bell pepper, diced

Combine all ingredients and mix well. Allow to chill at least one hour before serving. Serve cold. Makes 8 servings.

Each serving provides 200 calories, 5 g fat, 33 g carbohydrates, 450 mg sodium, 0 mg cholesterol, 8 g protein.

Source: Loma Linda University.

Chicken and White Bean Salad

8 ounces skinless, boneless   1 tablespoon olive oil
   chicken breast   1 teaspoon lemon juice
38-ounce can white beans   ¹/₄ cup balsamic vinegar
1 finely chopped red pepper   ¹/₂ teaspoon oregano
2 cloves garlic

Steam, boil, or microwave the chicken until cooked. Shred and place in a large bowl; add beans, red pepper, and garlic, and stir. Combine remaining ingredients together and pour over the chicken and beans and mix thoroughly. Best served chilled. Makes 6 servings.

Each serving provides: 238 calories, 6 g total fat, 31 g carbohydrate, 11 g dietary fiber, 17 g protein, 57 mg calcium, 3 mg iron.

Source: University of Utah, Nutrition Clinic.

Tuna Pasta Salad*

³/₄ cup elbow macaroni, uncooked
6.5-ounce can tuna, water-packed, drained
¹/₂ cup celery, thinly sliced
1 cup seedless red grapes, halved
3 tablespoons salad dressing, mayonnaise-type, reduced-calorie

Cook macaroni according to package directions, omitting salt. Drain. Toss macaroni, tuna, celery, and grapes together. Mix in salad dressing. Serve warm or chill until served. Makes 4 one-cup servings.

Menu Suggestions: Serve with broccoli spears, pumpernickel rolls, and ice milk topped with sliced strawberries.

Each serving provides: 195 calories, 2 g fat, trace saturated fatty acids, 13 mg cholesterol, 170 mg sodium.

Source: United States Department of Agriculture.

Broccoli Soup

1½ cups broccoli, chopped*
¼ cup celery, diced
¼ cup onion, chopped
1 cup chicken broth, unsalted
2 cups skim milk

2 tablespoons cornstarch
¼ teaspoon salt
Dash pepper
Dash ground thyme
¼ cup Swiss cheese, shredded

Place vegetables and broth in saucepan. Bring to boiling, reduce heat, cover, and cook until vegetables are tender—about 8 minutes. Mix milk, cornstarch, salt, pepper, and thyme; add to cooked vegetables. Cook, stirring constantly, until soup is slightly thickened and mixture just begins to boil. Remove from heat. Add cheese and stir until melted. Makes 4 one-cup servings.

*Note: A 10-ounce package of frozen chopped broccoli can be used in place of fresh broccoli. The soup will have about 120 calories and 260 mg of sodium per serving.

Each serving provides: 110 calories, 3 g fat, 2 g saturated fatty acids, 9 mg cholesterol, 250 mg sodium.

Source: United States Department of Agriculture.

Fish Stew*

1 pound cod or other white fish
1 tablespoon olive oil
1 onion, chopped
1 sweet green pepper, chopped
2 cloves garlic, chopped

1 teaspoon basil
28-ounce can whole tomatoes
  (low salt)
1 can tomato sauce (low salt)

Heat oil; add onion and green pepper, cook until soft; add garlic and basil, cook 1 minute. Add tomatoes and sauce; bring to boil, cut up tomatoes. Simmer 15 minutes. Cut fish into chunks and add to above; simmer until fish is cooked. Serve with rice. Makes 4 to 6 servings.

Source: Unpublished. From author's files.

White Bean Soup

$\frac{1}{2}$ pound dry navy beans, rinsed, or canned white beans, rinsed
1 tablespoon olive oil
2 celery stalks, cut up
1 carrot, sliced
1 onion
1 clove garlic
1 large can low-salt chicken broth
1 package frozen chopped spinach
$\frac{1}{2}$ cup elbow macaroni or other small pasta

Bring dry beans to boil in pan of water; boil 5 minutes. Remove from heat. Cover and let stand 1 hour. Drain. Stir fry celery, carrots, onion, and garlic in oil about 5 minutes. Add beans and chicken broth and bring to boil, cover and simmer until beans are tender—about 1 hour. Add spinach; boil then simmer until spinach is heated. Add cooked pasta.

Source: Unpublished. From author's files.

Split Pea Soup with Green Herbs

1 pound USA split peas, rinsed
2 quarts chicken stock or broth
1 large leek, chopped
1 tablespoon lemon juice
1 tablespoon sugar
$\frac{1}{8}$ teaspoon thyme
$\frac{1}{8}$ teaspoon marjoram
1 pinch nutmeg
3 tablespoons parsley, chopped
5 ounces spinach, washed and chopped, or frozen
Salt and pepper to taste

Combine split peas, chicken stock, leek, lemon juice, sugar, and spices. Cook slowly until peas are soft (45 to 60 minutes). Whisk or blend peas until pureed. Ten minutes before serving add spinach and parsley. Adjust consistency, season to taste with salt and pepper, enjoy! Serves 8 to 10.

Each serving provides: 235 calories, 3 g fat, 2 mg cholesterol, 1,278 mg sodium, 33 g carbohydrate, 3 g dietary fiber, 21 g protein.

Source: USA Dry Pea and Lentil Council, Moscow, Idaho.

Lentil Barley Soup

1 cup onion,chopped
1 cup celery, chopped
1 clove garlic, minced
$\frac{1}{4}$ cup vegetable oil
6 cups water
1 can (28 ounces) tomatoes or
    4 cups fresh tomatoes, diced
$\frac{3}{4}$ cup USA lentils, rinsed
1 cup shredded Swiss cheese,
    optional

$\frac{3}{4}$ cup pearl barley
6 vegetarian bouillon cubes
$\frac{1}{2}$ teaspoon dried rosemary,
    crushed
$\frac{1}{2}$ teaspoon dried oregano,
    crushed
$\frac{1}{4}$ teaspoon pepper
2 cups carrots, thinly sliced

In a large, heavy soup pot, cook the onions, celery, and garlic in hot oil until tender. Add the water, tomatoes, lentils, barley, bouillon cubes, rosemary, oregano, pepper, and carrots. Cook for 40 minutes, or until the barley, lentils, and carrots are tender. Top with Swiss cheese, if desired. Serves 10.

Each serving provides: 170 calories, 6 g fat, 0 mg cholesterol, 683 mg sodium, 26 g carbohydrate, 6 g dietary fiber, 5 g protein.

Source: USA Dry Pea and Lentil Council, Moscow, Idaho.

Vegetarian Split Pea Soup—Low Sodium

2 cups USA split peas, washed
2 quarts water
1 cup celery, sliced
$\frac{1}{2}$ cup onion, diced
1 cup carrots, chopped
1 cup potato, diced
1 clove garlic, minced

1 bay leaf
$\frac{1}{4}$ cup snipped fresh parsley
$\frac{1}{2}$ teaspoon crushed oregano
$\frac{1}{4}$ teaspoon crushed basil
1 teaspoon dried Italian seasoning
$\frac{1}{2}$ teaspoon salt
Pinch cayenne

Combine all ingredients in a Dutch oven. Bring to a boil. Reduce heat, cover, and simmer 1 hour or until split peas are cooked through. Remove bay leaf before serving. Makes 10 one-cup servings.

Each serving provides: 118 calories, less than 1 g fat, 139 mg sodium, 22 g carbohydrate, 5 g dietary fiber, 8 g protein.

Source: USA Dry Pea and Lentil Council, Moscow, Idaho.

Spicy Southwestern Chowder

2 slices bacon, chopped
1 medium onion, chopped
1 cup shredded carrots
  (about 2 medium)
1 to 2 jalapeño peppers,
  seeded and minced
2 cloves garlic, minced
1½ teaspoons chili powder
½ teaspoon ground cumin

3 cups low-fat milk
2 cups reduced-sodium
  chicken broth
3 cups cooked brown rice
16-ounce package frozen corn or
  17-ounce can corn, drained
6 large sourdough round rolls, hol-
  lowed out leaving ½-inch walls
Green onions for garnish

Cook bacon in Dutch oven over medium-high heat 5 to 7 minutes, stirring until bacon is crisp. Drain all but 1 tablespoon fat. Add onion, carrots, jalapeños, garlic, chili powder, and cumin. Cook 3 to 5 minutes, stirring constantly until onion is tender. Reduce heat to medium. Add milk, broth, rice, and corn. Cook, stirring, 10 to 12 minutes until mixture boils. Cook 1 minute more; remove from heat. Ladle into bread rounds. Garnish with green onions. Makes 6 servings.

Each serving provides: 590 calories, 7 g fat, 15 mg cholesterol, 780 mg sodium, 110 g carbohydrate, 5 g dietary fiber, 20 g protein.

Source: USA Rice Council, Houston, Texas.

Minestrone Soup*

½ cup uncooked regular
  or whole-wheat macaroni
16-ounce package frozen
  mixed vegetables

2 cups vegetable broth
15.5-ounce can kidney beans
16-ounce can tomatoes
2 tablespoons chopped parsley

Cook macaroni in boiling water for 10 minutes; drain. Chop vegetables; cook in vegetable broth for 15 minutes. Add beans, tomatoes, and macaroni. Add seasonings to taste. Makes 8 servings.

Each serving provides: 142 calories, 1.5 g fat, 26 g carbohydrate, 6 g fiber, 7 g protein, 38 mg calcium, 1.5 mg iron.

Source: University of Utah Nutrition Clinic.

Vegetable Soup*

1 8-ounce can low-salt tomato sauce	2 potatoes, sliced
1 cup water	1 zucchini, sliced
3 carrots, sliced	1 teaspoon basil
	Salt to taste

In saucepan, stir together tomato sauce, water, and salt. Add sliced vegetables and 1 teaspoon basil and bring to boil. Cook on low heat, covered, until vegetables are tender.

Source: Unpublished. From author's files.

Meatless Lentil Chili

2½ cups (1 pound) USA lentils, rinsed
5 cups water
1 packet (1 ounce) dry onion soup mix
1 can (16 ounces) tomatoes or tomato sauce
1½ teaspoons chili powder
½ teaspoon cumin

In a large saucepan, bring lentils and water to a boil. Add dry onion soup mix and simmer for 30 minutes. Add the rest of the ingredients and simmer 30 minutes longer. Serve over spaghetti, rice, or corn chips. Garnish with cheese. Chili can also be used on pizzas, in tacos, or as a dip. Serves 6 to 8.

Each serving provides: 210 calories, trace of fat, 333 mg cholesterol, 1,129 mg sodium, 40 g carbohydrate, 9 g dietary fiber, 14 g protein.

Source: USA Dry Pea and Lentil Council, Moscow, Idaho.

Northwest Lentil Chili

32-ounce can (4 cups) tomato juice ½ cup diced onion
2 cups diced, raw potato   2 tablespoons chili powder
15-ounce can garbanzo beans   2 teaspoons beef bouillon granules
1 cup USA lentils, washed   1 teaspoon crushed basil
1 cup diced carrots   2 cloves garlic, minced

Combine all ingredients in a Dutch oven and bring to a boil.
Reduce heat and simmer, covered, about 30 minutes or until
lentils are tender. Makes 10 one-cup servings.

Each serving provides: 152 calories, 1 g fat, 544 mg sodium,
29 g carbohydrate, 6 g dietary fiber, 9 g protein.

Source: USA Dry Pea and Lentil Council, Moscow, Idaho.

Rice Olé

1 cup each chopped onions   1 teaspoon each chili powder
   and green peppers   and garlic salt
½ cup celery, finely chopped   14.5-ounce can peeled
1 tablespoon butter   whole tomatoes, chopped
   or margarine   3 cups cooked rice

Combine onions, peppers, celery, and butter in 2½-quart
microwave-proof baking dish. Cover and cook on high 6 minutes.
Add seasonings, tomatoes, and rice; stir. Cover and cook on high
4 minutes. Let stand 5 minutes. Makes 6 servings.

Each serving provides: 128 calories, 2 g fat, 5 mg cholesterol,
489 mg sodium, 24 g carbohydrate, 3 g protein.

Source: USA Rice Council, Houston, Texas.

Spanish Rice

1½ cups uncooked brown rice
2½ cups water
2½ teaspoons salt seasoning
1 cup onion, chopped
½ cup green peppers
2 tablespoons corn oil

½ teaspoon garlic powder
½ cup tomatoes, diced,
   canned in puree
2 tablespoons tomato paste
½ teaspoon cumin
1 teaspoon salt

Cook rice in water with seasoning until tender (approximately 50 minutes). Sauté onions and green pepper in oil. Add garlic powder. Add remaining ingredients and cook for 5 minutes, stirring frequently. Add cooked rice. Mix well and simmer 3 to 4 minutes, stirring occasionally.

Source: Loma Linda University.

Dry Soybeans

Sort dry soybeans before cooking to remove any discolored, cracked, or shriveled beans. After sorting, measure beans and wash thoroughly. To soak and cook, follow the directions below. One cup of dry soybeans will yield about 2½ cups cooked beans.

To soak, use 4 cups of water for each cup of dry beans. To soak them quickly, boil beans 2 minutes, remove from heat, and let stand 1 hour. Or, if you prefer, boil beans 2 minutes and let them stand overnight in the refrigerator.

To boil, soak beans as directed above. Add 1 teaspoon salt for each cup of dry beans. Simmer, covered, in soaking water 2 to 3 hours until beans are tender. Add water, if necessary, during cooking. When done, the beans will be firm but tender, and not mealy. To reduce foaming, add 1 to 2 teaspoons oil or meat drippings to the cooking water.

Store dry soybeans in a cool, dry place. After cooking, store covered in the refrigerator. Cooked soybeans may be stored about 1 week.

Source: Utah State University Extension.

Bulgur

1. Wash wheat in cool water and discard water.

2. Cover wheat with 2 to 3 times as much water as wheat. Steam until water is absorbed and wheat is tender (about 35 to 40 minutes).

3. Spread cooked wheat thinly on cookie sheet and place in 200° F. oven to dry (leave door open). Wheat must be very dry in order to crack easily (this takes 2 to 3 hours). A food dehydrator may also be used.

4. Crack wheat in a mill, grinder, or blender. (This step is optional, but produces a finer kernel.)

5. Store in an air-tight container on shelf.

6. Re-hydrate for recipes calling for cooked wheat or cooked bulgur by adding twice as much liquid as bulgur and boiling 5 to 10 minutes. Bulgur will approximately double in volume.

Source: Utah State University Extension, Salt Lake County.

Chicken Dijon*

1/4 cup Dijon-style mustard
1/4 cup low-fat or fat-free mayonnaise
2 chicken breasts (skinned, halved)
1 cup cornflake crumbs
1/3 cup Parmesan cheese

Blend mayonnaise and mustard and coat chicken; roll in crumbs. Cover with cheese and bake at 325° F. for 1 hour. Serves 2.

Source: Unpublished. From author's files.

Curry Chicken*

1 pound boneless, skinless chicken breasts or thighs, chunked
1 tablespoon olive oil
1 onion, chopped
4 cloves garlic, sliced thin

2 teaspoons curry powder or more if you like it a little spicier
$1/4$ teaspoon ground ginger
$1/8$ teaspoon salt
$1/2$ cup chopped tomatoes
$1/3$ cup water

Sauté chicken in oil until browned all over. Put chicken in bowl; pat up excess oil with paper towels, and keep warm. Lower heat and add onion and garlic to pan. Cook, stirring frequently, until lightly browned and soft. Stir in curry powder, ginger, and salt; cook 1 minute. Stir in tomato and water; cook 1 minute more. Add chicken; bring to boiling. Lower heat; cover and simmer until chicken is cooked and no pink remains. Serve over rice, with chopped nuts, parsley, raisins, or low-fat yogurt.

Source: Unpublished. From author's files.

Italian Chicken*

4 chicken breast halves, skinned
$1/2$ cup onion, chopped
$1/2$ medium green pepper, chopped
2 8-ounce cans no-salt-added tomato sauce

$1/2$ teaspoon oregano leaves
$1/4$ teaspoon basil leaves
$1/8$ teaspoon garlic powder
$1/8$ teaspoon salt

Brown chicken in hot frying pan. Mix the rest of the ingredients together and pour the mixture over chicken. Heat the mixture until it boils, then reduce the heat, cover, and cook over low heat until chicken is tender, about 45 minutes. Makes 4 servings (1 serving is 1 breast-half and $1/2$ cup sauce).

Each serving provides: 190 calories, 2 g fat, 70 mg cholesterol, 180 mg sodium.

Source: United States Department of Agriculture.

Chicken-Style A La King

1 12.5-ounce can Worthington
    Fri-Chik, drained (reserve liquid)
½ cup skim milk
2 tablespoons all-purpose flour
½ cup frozen peas

½ cup green peppers, diced
2 tablespoons pimento
½ cup mushrooms, diced
1 tablespoon seasoning salt
$\frac{1}{16}$ teaspoon turmeric

Drain Fri-Chick, saving liquid. Dice Fri-Chik; set aside. Add enough milk to Fri-Chik liquid to make 2 cups. Combine liquid, flour, and remaining milk; cook over medium heat until thickened. Add diced Fri-Chik, peas, peppers, pimento, mushrooms, and seasonings to sauce. Serve hot over toast or rice.

Source: Loma Linda University.

Turkey Casserole

½ cup chopped onion
½ cup chopped celery
1–2 tablespoons olive oil
1 can whole cranberries

2 cups cooked, chopped turkey
6-ounce package wild rice
    or wild rice/white rice mix
3 tablespoons cooking wine

Prepare rice according to package directions. Cook onion and celery in oil until tender. Stir in 1 can whole cranberries and 3 tablespoons white cooking wine. Stir in turkey and rice. Put in baking dish. Bake covered at 350° F. for 35 to 45 minutes. Stir.

Source: Unpublished. From author's files.

Broiled Sesame Fish

For a quick, low-fat main dish, try this fish recipe. It takes about 15 minutes to prepare and contains very little fat.

1 pound cod fillets, fresh or frozen	$\frac{1}{8}$ teaspoon salt
1 teaspoon margarine, melted	Dash pepper
1 tablespoon lemon juice	1 tablespoon sesame seed
1 teaspoon dried tarragon leaves	1 tablespoon parsley, chopped

Thaw frozen fish in refrigerator overnight or defrost briefly in a microwave oven. Cut fish into four portions. Place fish on a broiler pan lined with aluminum foil. Brush margarine over fish. Mix lemon juice, tarragon leaves, salt, and pepper. Pour over fish. Sprinkle sesame seeds evenly over fish. Broil until fish flakes easily when tested with a fork—about 12 minutes. Garnish each serving with parsley. Makes 4 2.5-ounce servings.

Each serving provides: 110 calories, 3 g fat, trace saturated fatty acids, 46 mg cholesterol, 155 mg sodium.

Source: United States Department of Agriculture.

Fish Parmesan

1 $\frac{1}{2}$ pounds filleted fish	$\frac{1}{2}$ cup skim-milk grated
garlic salt, pepper	mozzarella cheese
$\frac{1}{2}$ teaspoon oregano	2 tablespoons Parmesan cheese
8-ounce jar marinara sauce	

Season fish with garlic salt, pepper, and oregano. Put fish in baking dish. Pour marinara sauce over it. Sprinkle with cheeses and bake at 425° F. for 15 minutes. Serves 4.

Source: Unpublished. From author's files.

Vegetable Quesadillas*

1 red pepper, raw
1 yellow pepper, raw
4 scallions
1 carrot, raw
8 pieces iceberg lettuce
2 cups tomatoes, chopped

8 ounces mozzarella
  part-skim cheese
1 cup plain nonfat yogurt
4 tablespoons hot picante salsa
4 corn tortillas

Chop the vegetables and mix together. Combine salsa and yogurt, set aside. Arrange vegetables on the corn tortillas, top with cheese, and fold in half. Microwave on high for about 40 seconds. Top with lettuce and salsa/yogurt mixture. Makes 4 servings.

Each serving provides: 313 calories, 30% DV fat, 33 mg cholesterol, 524 mg sodium, 39% DV carbohydrate, 31% DV protein, 618 mg calcium, 2 mg iron.

Source: University of Utah Nutrition Clinic.

Brown Rice Black Bean Burrito

1 tablespoon vegetable oil
1 medium onion, chopped
2 cloves garlic, minced
1 1/2 teaspoons chili powder
1/2 teaspoon cumin
3 cups cooked brown rice
15- to 16-ounce can black beans,
  drained and rinsed

11-ounce can corn, drained
6 (8-inch) flour tortillas
3/4 cup (6 ounces) shredded
  reduced-fat cheddar cheese
2 green onions, thinly sliced
1/4 cup plain low-fat yogurt
1/4 cup prepared salsa

Heat oil in large skillet over medium-high heat until hot. Add onion, garlic, chili powder, and cumin. Sauté 3 to 5 minutes until onion is tender. Add rice, beans, and corn; cook, stirring 2 to 3 minutes until mixture is thoroughly heated. Remove from heat. Spoon 1/2 cup rice mixture down center of each tortilla. Top each with 2 tablespoons cheese, 1 tablespoon green onion, and 1 tablespoon yogurt; roll up, top with 1 tablespoon salsa. Makes 6 servings.

Each serving provides: 456 calories, 9 g fat, 10 mg cholesterol, 591 mg sodium, 73 g carbohydrate, 6 g dietary fiber, 23 g protein.

Source: USA Rice Council, Houston, Texas.

Shrimp Pita

¾ cup olive oil
½ cup red wine vinegar
2 medium onions, chopped,
   divided
2 cloves garlic, minced,
   divided
2 teaspoons Italian seasoning,
   divided
1 pound medium shrimp, peeled
   and deveined

2 medium-sized red or green
   bell peppers, julienned
4 cups fresh spinach leaves,
   stems removed and torn
3 cups cooked brown rice
1 teaspoon salt
½ teaspoon ground black pepper
3 pieces pita bread (6 inches)
   each cut in half

Combine oil, vinegar, ½ cup chopped onion, 1 clove garlic, and 1 teaspoon Italian seasoning in large bowl. Add shrimp; stir until well coated. Cover and refrigerate 4 hours or overnight. Thoroughly drain shrimp; discard marinade. Heat large skillet over medium-high heat until hot. Add shrimp, remaining onion, bell peppers, spinach, and remaining 1 clove garlic; sauté 3 to 5 minutes or until shrimp is no longer pink and spinach is wilted. Add rice, remaining 1 teaspoon Italian seasoning, salt, and pepper. Cook and stir 2 to 3 minutes or until flavors are well blended. To serve, fill each pita with ½- to ¾-cup rice. Makes 6 servings.

Each serving provides: 296 calories, 6 g fat, 61 mg cholesterol, 677 mg sodium, 47 g carbohydrate, 6 g dietary fiber, 14 g protein.

Source: USA Rice Council, Houston, Texas.

Beef and Vegetable Stir-Fry

³/₄ pound (12 ounces) beef
   round steak, boneless
1 teaspoon vegetable oil
¹/₂ cup carrots, sliced
¹/₄ cup celery, sliced
¹/₂ cup onion, sliced
1 tablespoon soy sauce

¹/₈ teaspoon garlic powder
Dash pepper
2 cups zucchini squash,
   cut in thin strips
1 tablespoon cornstarch
¹/₄ cup water

Trim all fat from steak. Slice steak across the grain into thin strips about ¹/₈-inch wide and 3 inches long. (Partially frozen meat is easier to slice.) Heat oil in frying pan. Add beef strips and stir fry over high heat, turning pieces constantly, until beef is no longer red—about 3 to 5 minutes. Reduce heat. Add carrots, celery, onion, and seasonings. Cover and cook until carrots are slightly tender—3 to 4 minutes. Add squash; cook until vegetables are tender-crisp—3 to 4 minutes. Mix cornstarch and water until smooth; add slowly to beef mixture, stirring constantly. Cook until thickened and vegetables are coated with a thin glaze. Makes 4 ³/₄-cup servings. You may substitute 12 ounces of raw chicken for the beef if desired.

Each serving provides: 145 calories, 4 g fat, 1 g saturated fatty acids, 44 mg cholesterol, 300 mg sodium.

With chicken, each serving provides: 140 calories, 2 g fat, trace saturated fatty acids, 51 mg cholesterol, 320 mg sodium.

Source: United States Department of Agriculture.

Spicy Steak Strips

³/₄ pound beef round steak,
  boneless
¹/₂ cup celery, sliced
¹/₂ cup onion, chopped
1 tablespoon flour
16-ounce can tomatoes
¹/₂ cup water
2 tablespoons parsley,
  chopped

1 tablespoon Worcestershire
  sauce
¹/₂ teaspoon ginger root,
  minced
¹/₄ teaspoon salt
¹/₈ teaspoon ground cloves
¹/₈ teaspoon red pepper flakes
1 bay leaf

Trim all fat from steak. Slice across the grain diagonally into thin strips. (It is easier to slice steak into thin strips if it is partially frozen.) Heat nonstick frying pan. Cook steak, celery, and onion until steak is browned. Drain off fat. Stir flour into beef mixture. Add remaining ingredients. Bring to a boil; reduce heat, cover, and cook over low heat for 40 minutes or until meat is tender. Remove bay leaf. Serve over noodles or rice. Makes 4 half-cup servings.

Each serving provides (not including noodles or rice): 140 calories, 3 g fat, 1 g saturated fatty acids, 43 mg cholesterol, 245 mg sodium.

Source: United States Department of Agriculture.

Bagel Pizza

1 bagel

On each half place:
    1 tablespoon pre-made pizza sauce
    1¹/₂ ounces mozzarella cheese
    sliced tomatoes
    mushrooms
    red onions

Bake at 400° F. for 4 to 5 minutes.

Source: Unpublished. From author's files.

Homemade Pasta Sauce

3 cloves garlic, crushed
2 tablespoons olive oil
1–2 cans (28 ounces) crushed
   tomatoes or fresh
   skinned tomatoes

3 tablespoons chopped
   fresh basil
1 small zucchini or yellow
   squash, sliced
Fresh or canned mushrooms

Sauté garlic, mushrooms, and zucchini in oil. Add tomatoes; cook uncovered until slightly thickened. Stir in basil.

Source: Unpublished: From author's files.

Chili Bean Dip

15-ounce can kidney beans
3 tablespoons drained bean liquid
1 tablespoon vinegar
1 teaspoon chili powder

$\frac{1}{8}$ teaspoon ground cumin
2 teaspoons onion, grated
2 teaspoons parsley, chopped

Drain kidney beans; save liquid. Place drained beans, bean liquid, vinegar, and seasonings in blender. Blend until smooth. Remove mixture from blender. Stir in onion and parsley. Chill thoroughly. Serve with crisp vegetable sticks. Makes about $1\frac{1}{3}$ cups.

Each tablespoon serving provides: 15 calories, trace fat, trace saturated fatty acids, 0 mg cholesterol, 55 mg sodium.

Source: United States Department of Agriculture.

Hot "N" Spicy Seasoning

$\frac{1}{4}$ cup paprika
2 tablespoons oregano
2 teaspoons chili powder
1 teaspoon garlic powder

1 teaspoon black pepper
$\frac{1}{2}$ teaspoon red pepper
$\frac{1}{2}$ teaspoon dry mustard

Mix all of the above in a bowl. Store in airtight container.

This seasoning tastes good on meat, poultry, or fish. Instead of salt, sprinkle some on the food and then cook it as you usually do. Or, mix some with plain breadcrumbs and then coat the meat with the crumbs. If you like it very spicy, use more.

Source: National Institute of Health.

Cheese Sauce for Broccoli and Cauliflower

4 tablespoons margarine or butter
4 tablespoons flour
2 cups skim milk
1 cup low-fat or non-fat grated cheese—any yellow cheese

Steam broccoli and cauliflower until tender.

Melt margarine or butter in frying pan. Add flour and stir. Add milk; stir on low heat until thickened. Add grated cheese; stir until melted.

Put cauliflower and broccoli in baking dish; pour cheese sauce on top and bake at 300° F. for 30 minutes.

Source: Unpublished. From author's files.

Fruit Smoothie*

1½ cups skim or 1 percent milk
6-ounce can frozen orange or other juice (softened)
1 cup water
1½ teaspoons vanilla extract

Pour milk in large bowl or blender. Add other ingredients and whisk or blend until foamy. Serve immediately.

Source: University of Illinois at Urbana-Champaign.

Granola*

6 cups rolled oats
1 cup wheat germ
1 cup unprocessed bran

1 cup roasted sunflower seeds
1 cup roasted almonds, chopped
1½ cups raisins

Mix above ingredients together and store in an air-tight container. If desired, cereal can be toasted on a greased cookie sheet for 20 minutes in a 300° F. oven. Makes approximately 20 half-cup servings.

Each serving provides: 246 calories, 34% DV fat, 0 mg cholesterol, 55 mg sodium, 51% DV carbohydrate, 15% DV protein, 45 mg calcium, 3 mg iron.

Source: University of Utah Nutrition Clinic.

Blender Pancakes

1 cup wheat, uncooked

1 1/2 cups milk*

1 egg

3 tablespoons sugar

1 teaspoon salt

1 tablespoon baking powder

2 tablespoons oil

Combine wheat and 1 cup of milk in blender. Blend on high for 1 minute. Add remaining ingredients and blend until smooth. Cook on hot griddle. Serve with favorite topping.

*Dry milk may be substituted. Add 4 tablespoons non-instant powdered milk or 1/2 cup instant milk powder to wheat. Then use the same amount of water as called for with fresh milk. Makes 6 to 8 servings.

Each serving provides: 175 calories, 6 g fat, 33 mg cholesterol, 453 mg sodium, 24 g carbohydrate, 1 g dietary fiber, 6 g protein.

Source: Utah State University Extension, Salt Lake County.

Sweet Gingercrisp

$\frac{1}{3}$ cup maple syrup
$\frac{1}{4}$ cup lemon juice
3 tablespoons water
1 teaspoon vanilla extract
4 cups sliced unpeeled apples
3 cups cooked brown rice
Vegetable cooking spray
2 tablespoons all-purpose flour

2 tablespoons brown
   sugar, packed
1 teaspoon allspice
2 tablespoons butter
   or margarine
$\frac{3}{4}$ cup coarsely crushed
   gingersnap cookies (about 10)
1 cup nonfat vanilla yogurt,
   divided

Combine maple syrup, lemon juice, water, and vanilla in large bowl. Stir in apples and rice. Spoon into casserole dish coated with cooking spray. Combine flour, brown sugar, and allspice in small bowl; cut in butter until crumbly. Stir in gingersnaps and sprinkle over apples and rice. Bake covered in 400° F. oven 35 minutes. Remove cover, bake 10 minutes more or until top is golden brown and apples are tender. Serve warm, topping each serving with 1 tablespoon yogurt. Makes 8 servings.

Each serving provides: 268 calories, 5 g fat, 12 mg cholesterol, 210 mg sodium, 52 g carbohydrate, 2 g dietary fiber, 4 g protein.

Source: USA Rice Council, Houston, Texas.

Apple Crisp

4 cups tart apples, pared, sliced
$1/4$ cup water
1 tablespoon lemon juice
$1/4$ cup brown sugar, packed
$1/4$ cup whole-wheat flour

$1/4$ cup old-fashioned rolled oats
$1/2$ teaspoon ground cinnamon
$1/4$ teaspoon ground nutmeg
3 tablespoons margarine

Place apples in 8- by 8- by 2-inch baking pan. Mix water and lemon juice; pour over apples. Mix sugar, flour, oats, and spices. Add margarine to dry mixture; mix until crumbly. Sprinkle crumbly mixture evenly over apples. Bake at 350° F. until apples are tender and topping is lightly browned, about 40 minutes. Makes 4 half-cup servings.

Each serving provides: 235 calories, 9 g fat, 2 g saturated fatty acids, 0 mg cholesterol, 105 mg sodium.

Source: United States Department of Agriculture.

Johnnycake

$1 1/4$ cups flour
$3/4$ cup cornmeal
2 tablespoons sugar
2 teaspoons baking powder
$1/2$ teaspoon salt

1 cup milk
$1/4$ cup cooking oil
4 tablespoons molasses or syrup
2 eggs

Preheat oven to 350° F. Grease an 8- or 9-inch square pan. Combine flour, cornmeal, sugar, baking powder, and salt. Stir in milk, oil, molasses, and eggs, mixing until dry. Bake 20 to 25 minutes. Makes 1 loaf.

Source: LDS Church Archives.

Fruit Bran Muffins*

2½ cups bran cereal
1½ cups skim milk
4 egg whites
1 tablespoon vanilla
2 cups flour

½ cup brown sugar
1½ teaspoons cinnamon
2 tablespoons baking powder
¾ teaspoon baking soda
2 cups fresh or frozen fruit or
    dried cranberries or cherries

Preheat oven to 325° F. Combine cereal, milk, egg whites, and vanilla. Stir together flour, brown sugar, cinnamon, baking powder, and baking soda. Combine dry and wet mixtures. Fold in fruit. Spoon into paper-lined muffin tins. Bake for 30 minutes.

Each serving provides: 141 calories, 4% DV fat, 82% DV carbohydrates, 14% DV protein.

Source: University of Utah Nutrition Clinic.

Pumpkin Cupcakes

1½ cups whole-wheat flour
1 cup all-purpose flour
¾ cup sugar
2 tablespoons baking powder
2 teaspoons ground cinnamon
½ teaspoon ground nutmeg
¼ teaspoon salt

3 eggs, slightly beaten
1 cup skim milk
½ cup vegetable oil
1 cup canned pumpkin
¾ cup raisins, chopped
1 tablespoon vanilla

Preheat oven to 350° F. Place 24 paper baking cups in muffin tins. Mix dry ingredients thoroughly. Mix remaining ingredients; add to dry ingredients. Stir until dry ingredients are barely moistened. Fill paper cups two-thirds full. Bake about 20 minutes or until toothpick inserted in center comes out clean. Remove from muffin tins and cool on rack. Freeze cupcakes that will not be eaten in the next few days. Makes 24 cupcakes.

Each cupcake serving provides: 140 calories, 5 g fat, 1 g saturated fatty acids, 27 mg cholesterol, 130 mg sodium.

Source: United States Department of Agriculture.

Oatmeal Applesauce Cookies

1 cup all-purpose flour
1 teaspoon baking powder
1 teaspoon ground allspice
$1/_4$ teaspoon salt
$1/_2$ cup margarine

$1/_2$ cup sugar
2 egg whites
2 cups rolled oats, quick-cooking
1 cup unsweetened applesauce
$1/_2$ cup raisins, chopped

Preheat oven to 375° F. Grease baking sheet. Mix flour, baking powder, allspice, and salt. Beat margarine and sugar until creamy. Add egg whites; beat well. Add dry ingredients. Stir in oats, applesauce, and raisins. Mix well. Drop by level tablespoonfuls onto baking sheet. Bake 11 minutes or until edges are lightly browned. Cool on rack. Makes about 5 dozen cookies.

Each cookie serving provides: 45 calories, 2 g fat, trace saturated fatty acids, 0 mg cholesterol, 35 mg sodium.

Source: United States Department of Agriculture.

Zucchini Bread

1 cup whole-wheat flour
1 cup all-purpose flour
$1^1/_2$ teaspoons baking powder
1 teaspoon ground cinnamon
$1/_4$ teaspoon baking soda
$1/_4$ teaspoon salt

3 egg whites
$1/_2$ cup sugar
$1/_3$ cup vegetable oil
$1^1/_2$ teaspoons vanilla
2 cups zucchini squash, coarsely
     shredded, lightly packed

Preheat oven to 350° F. Grease 9- by 5- by 3-inch loaf pan. Mix dry ingredients, except sugar. Beat egg whites until frothy. Add sugar, oil, and vanilla. Continue beating for 3 minutes. Stir in zucchini; mix lightly. Add dry ingredients. Mix just until dry ingredients are moistened. Pour into loaf pan. Bake 40 minutes or until toothpick inserted in center comes out clean. Cool on rack. Remove from pan after 10 minutes. To serve, cut into 18 slices about $1/_2$-inch thick. Makes 1 loaf.

Each slice serving provides: 110 calories, 4 g fat, 1 g saturated fatty acids, 0 mg cholesterol, 90 mg sodium.

Source: United States Department of Agriculture.

Bran Apple Bars

Apples and bran cereal add dietary fiber. Using egg whites in place of a whole egg keeps cholesterol to a trace.

1 cup whole-bran cereal*	¼ teaspoon ground nutmeg
½ cup skim milk	⅓ cup margarine
1 cup flour	½ cup brown sugar, packed
1 teaspoon baking powder	2 egg whites
½ teaspoon ground cinnamon	1 cup apple, pared, chopped

Preheat oven to 350° F. Grease 9- by 9-inch baking pan. Soak bran in milk until milk is absorbed. Mix dry ingredients thoroughly. Beat margarine and sugar until creamy. Add egg whites; beat well. Stir in apples and bran mixture. Add dry ingredients; mix well. Pour into pan. Bake 30 minutes or until a toothpick inserted in center comes out clean. Cool on rack. Cut into 16 bars.

* Note: Check the nutrition label of cereals for sodium content. Some whole-bran cereals contain almost twice as much sodium as others.

Each bar serving provides: 110 calories, 4 g fat, 1 g saturated fatty acids, trace cholesterol, 110 mg sodium.

Source: United States Department of Agriculture.

——— 6 ———

THE DIET SOLUTION FOR ALL AGES

*"Each of us has agency; each is free to choose. Nothing
can free us spiritually more than obedience—obedience
to the laws, to the Lord. Nothing is more liberating spiritually than the worthiness which is maintained, and at
times perhaps must be reclaimed, through repentance. We
need to keep the Word of Wisdom (that is the key to revelation, to treasures of knowledge, even hidden treasures)."*

—Boyd K. Packer

CHILDREN

One of the major worries of health experts is the growing
number of overweight and obese children. And because
overweight children tend to become overweight adults, the
problem can mean a lifetime of poor health. Children need
the same nutrients as adults, just in smaller sized servings. A
study cited in the journal *Pediatrics* found that only one percent of American children get all the nutrients recommended
in the Food Guide Pyramid. At the same time, the number
of overweight children in the United States has gone from
5 percent to 11 percent over the last decade.[34]

Ask your pediatrician about your child's nutritional
needs, but remember that you are the example for good or

bad eating habits. The food guidelines in the Word of Wisdom were meant to make children healthier. Introduce your children to a wide variety of fruits and vegetables. That way, if they do not like one kind, chances are you can find substitutes that provide the same vitamins and other nutrients. For example, if they will not eat sweet potatoes, carrots will do just fine. I have included in appendixes A and B a list of fruits and vegetables and their vitamins. Get children used to whole grains as soon as your doctor says they are ready. Children over six years old need three servings of milk a day. If they are under two they need whole milk. Children also need more grains and vegetables than they are getting. (Think the middle range of the Food Guide Pyramid. They do not need a lot of meat. Two servings of protein a day is right for them. Too often a hot dog is a typical meat for a child. A small, two-ounce hot dog has *four teaspoons* of fat. That's 16 grams of fat. They do not need other high-fat foods or a lot of sugar either. Get children into the habit of drinking plenty of water, especially after they come in from play. Better still, send them out to play with a water bottle.

On the following page is the USDA's new Food Guide Pyramid for Young Children ages two to six.

Children are notorious for their eating likes and dislikes—ranging from not wanting foods to touch each other on the plate to rejecting or accepting certain foods based on color. Younger children especially like to have their food "dressed up." The more appealing you make the meal look, the more likely you are to get them to eat it. There is much you can do to influence your children's eating habits and make their meals and snacks enjoyable and healthy. Eating as a family and spending a relaxing, positive mealtime together can make a big difference. If you are not eating out as often and if you are avoiding fast-food restaurants most of the time, you are already making progress toward feeding your family healthier meals.

Food Guide Pyramid for Young Children

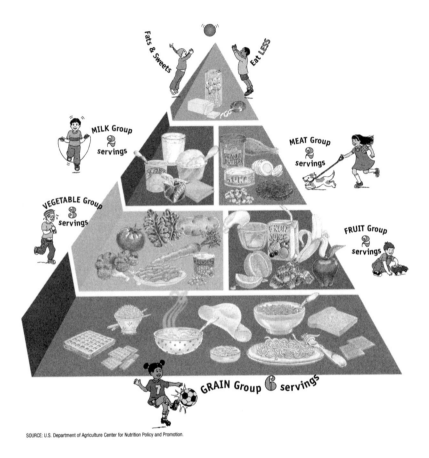

SOURCE: U.S. Department of Agriculture Center for Nutrition Policy and Promotion.

Snacks are an important supplement to your children's meals. Because they cannot eat a lot at once, children get hungry between meals and need something to eat. Healthy snacks could include graham crackers, applesauce, peanut butter crackers or peanut butter toast, and frozen fruit bars. You can puree your own fruit or use juice and freeze it in bars. In this way you can cut back significantly on the amount of sugar that store-bought bars contain. Try giving your children cheese slices with a fruit cup or a fig cookie and milk. My son is happy after school with a plate of sliced apples and some carrot and celery sticks, especially if I dress them up a bit. Celery with a little peanut butter and a few raisins on top becomes "ants on a log" and is thereby much more popular. Sometimes I fix him and his friends plain popped corn. Another good snack is a homemade cereal mix of wheat, corn, and oat squares with some nuts and bite-sized pretzels mixed in. The store-bought, pre-mixed kind has much more salt. You can also melt cheese on whole-wheat or regular tortillas and cut into wedges. If your children are old enough, let them make their own "smoothies" with fruit or fruit juice and skim milk or low-fat yogurt. Add a little vanilla extract for flavoring. They can also make their own pizzas using a whole-wheat English muffin topped with pizza sauce and a slice of cheese toasted under the broiler for a minute or two.

Like you, children ought to be able to have candy, cake, and cookies once in a while. But these should be eaten in small amounts and should not replace nutritious foods. Be careful that your attitude about these foods does not make them seem "extra special" and therefore a lot more desirable and somehow better. Include children in meal planning, discussing healthy choices with them. Let them help make up the shopping list and even help with the shopping. Preparing part of the meal is another way that children can feel they are making a contribution to a healthier family. Get a children's cookbook. It is my personal opinion that the more children understand about how proper nutrition and exercise help their bodies, the less likely they will be as they get older to take substances that will hurt their bodies. Ask your children's teachers what is being taught about nutrition. If nothing is being done, volunteer to come in for a few weeks and talk about healthy foods with the class.

Exercise is another area health experts worry about, because children are getting less and less of it. One of the best things you can do is cut the amount of time your

children watch TV. Another thing you can do is spend some
time exercising as a family—bike riding, skating, hiking,
holding a family obstacle course or a family Olympics. Talk
over with them what happens when they exercise—explain
what their heart, lungs, and muscles are doing. This will
help them realize how wonderful their bodies are. From an
early age, children are taught in family home evening
lessons and in church not to drink coffee, tea, or alcohol and
not to use tobacco. The teaching of the Word of Wisdom can
also be expanded to include the nutritional guidelines of the
Word of Wisdom. Young children are just as capable as
adults when it comes to learning what foods are good for
their bodies.

TEENS

The pressure on teenage girls to look like the thin women
they see in movies, on TV, and in magazines can be over-
whelming. Vomiting after eating, taking diet pills, and skipping meals are common ways for teenage girls to try to lose
weight. Unnecessary dieting at this age can retard growth
and increase the risk of diseases later in life. The National
Centers for Disease Control and Prevention conducted a
survey of over 11,000 high school students and found that
more than a third of the girls considered themselves overweight. Almost half of the girls said they were on a diet.[35]
The October 1999 issue of *Pediatrics* carried a report docu-
menting that young people are turning to cigarettes as a
way to lose weight.[36] What really throws young girls is the
onset of puberty when fat suddenly appears, or so it seems.
Girls go from 12 percent body fat before adolescence to as
much as 25 percent afterwards.[37]

Some teenagers do need to lose weight, and obesity is a
serious health risk for adolescents and teens. An article in
U.S. News & World Report points to a 70 percent increase in
the rate of obesity among young adults.[38] High blood

pressure and cholesterol, diabetes, strokes, and heart disease can start early in teens who are severely overweight. Compounding the problem is a cutback in the frequency of physical education classes in high school and an increase in the number of high schools offering fast foods such as hamburgers and fries for lunch.[39]

There is a right way and a wrong way to diet, and too many teenagers choose the wrong way. It is very difficult to get kids to eat healthy foods, especially when they spend so little time at home. High-fat foods from convenience stores and fast-food restaurants are typical fare for teenagers. Make sure that you have at least one meal together as a family every day and plan it out so that it is nutritionally balanced. Teenagers need three servings of milk/milk products a day. The Food Guide Pyramid suggests that girls get about 2,200 calories and boys get 2,800 calories a day to maintain a healthy weight. Boys can eat from the high end of the recommended number of servings in the pyramid and girls can eat from the middle range if they do not need to lose weight. It's not too late to get your older children involved in meal planning, shopping, and preparation. Like the rest of us, teenagers are not getting enough exercise. Do whatever you can to encourage your young people to be active, and set the example. When they are about to get on the phone, recommend they meet their friend for a "walk and talk" instead. Suggest their dating activities include sports.

Teenage boys are often interested in weight training. The best kind of weight training diet is following the Food Guide Pyramid. They do not need to bulk up on protein to build muscles. Nor do they need protein drinks or energy drinks. Sports nutritionists recommend athletes eat high-starch meals that include pasta, breads, cereals, fruits, and vegetables for energy about three hours or more before competitions.[40] Talk to your children about the Word of Wisdom. They may feel that if they are not drinking, smoking, or taking drugs that they are doing all that is required. Praise them for trying to do what is right, but point out that the Word of Wisdom is about more than alcohol, tobacco, tea, and coffee.

MIDDLE AGE

Middle-agers are at a critical point. But it is not too late to make positive changes in diet and lifestyle that will affect your health and quality of life in your senior years. Baby boomers are a large population bloc that will be facing rising health care costs and medical challenges. You will want to be able to "run and not be weary" as the years progress (D&C 89:20).

For women and men, this is a frustrating time as far as our bodies are concerned. I have finally come to realize that sooner or later the genes win. Not many people are "naturally fat," but where their fat is stored and a person's size and shape are genetically determined. This does not mean you should let yourself go because you don't like how you look and decide there is nothing you can do about it. Your appearance and your health can be greatly improved by diet, exercise, and attitude.

The women in my family have what we call "The Carver Curse." It is a pear-shaped body, with heavy emphasis on bottom, hips, and thighs. The legs aren't so great either—no tapering from the knees down and no dainty ankles. There is a limit to what exercise can do. My pre-determined shape became most apparent in middle age, and that's that. I have had to change my attitude. Instead of focusing on the negative physical attributes I think I inherited, I am learning to appreciate the positive attributes—physical, mental, and spiritual—that have been passed down to me. They are considerable and I am grateful.

According to the article in *U.S. News & World Report*, men and women in their fifties are more likely to be obese than at any other time in their lives. It makes a difference where the extra fat is located. Fat around the midsection is most dangerous because it surrounds the internal organs. Although men are more likely to store fat here, menopausal women get a wider waistline too. This means they also are more susceptible to diabetes and heart disease. Menopause poses other problems: Women in particular lose bone mass, making them at risk for osteoporosis, known as brittle bone disease. Colon cancer becomes more prevalent in women over forty. The decrease in estrogen, loss of muscle, and slower metabolism means women typically gain weight, usually five pounds, but often more. If you are not active, the muscle loss can be substantial over time and so can the weight gain.[41] This is the time when it's more important than ever to eat a nutritionally balanced diet with lots of fiber, to cut back on salt, to do aerobic exercise several times a week and strength training two or three times a week. Chapter 13 gives the details. You may find you have to exercise more and eat less than you did when you were younger to control your weight. You may also need to take a calcium supplement. You should discuss that and the question of hormone replacement therapy with your doctor. Phytoestrogens are natural plant sources of estrogens. They do not supply enough to make up for the loss during menopause, but ongoing research indicates they *may* help fight osteoporosis, breast cancer, and heart disease. Soy products are the best source of phytoestrogens.[42]

Middle age need not be looked upon as "the beginning of the end." It can be a time of good health, with more freedom, more financial security, and more opportunities for learning and service.

SENIORS

Seniors need to continue the good eating and exercise habits that they started in middle age, if not younger. It is no time to stop. In fact, it is the worst time to stop. Weightlifting can continue to halt osteoporosis. Walking and other weight-bearing exercise can help maintain muscle mass and keep the body strong. If you have not exercised in the past, start now, if your doctor gives the OK. Seniors need to reduce the amount of saturated fat and sodium in their diet and increase the amount of fiber. Just adding split peas or lentils to your favorite soup will help. So will eating more fruits, vegetables, and whole grains. It is important to get enough calcium and vitamin D. A balanced diet based on the Word of Wisdom and the Food Guide Pyramid will contribute to overall better health, despite the problems associated with the aging process. Older people sometimes find they have lost their sense of taste, so they add more salt. Try other seasonings instead. The sense of thirst can diminish as well, so keep drinking water and juices, even if you don't feel thirsty. Sometimes teeth and gum problems interfere with eating raw fruits and vegetables. Cooked fruits and vegetables still have fiber, as do cereals and breads made from whole grains. Eating alone can be depressing, but avoid skipping meals. Because cooking for one or two may seem like too much work, seniors often buy prepared foods, which can contain a lot of salt and fat or lack enough nutrition. Keep some food on hand to supplement packaged food. Whenever possible, make your own meals and enough extra to freeze for more meals later. Snacking is a good alternative for seniors with smaller appetites. Many seniors eat out often. It is important to choose restaurants and meals carefully, avoiding heavy sauces and gravies and fried foods. Have desserts only occasionally. Find restaurants that offer senior portions, or take home leftovers. Homebound seniors can arrange for home-delivered meals. The service typically supplies one meal a day and provides one-third of the nutritional requirements for the day. Check with your area agency on aging or your local senior citizen center.

Be Physically Active

If you are physically active your health will improve regardless of your age. Talk to your doctor first about what kind of exercise is right for you. I interviewed a friend of mine, Sarah Goodlin, M.D., who specializes in geriatric medicine at LDS Hospital in Salt Lake City, Utah. She had some interesting observations from her years of treating senior citizens. Most of her patients' weight problems fall into the unhealthy extremes of too heavy or too thin. Those older adults on the too-heavy side do not realize that they need fewer calories. She says that for every decade after thirty years of age you need one hundred fewer calories per day. At age sixty or seventy, people need three hundred or four hundred fewer calories per day than when they were thirty, but they tend to keep eating the same amount. Being overweight exacerbates the problems of old age. According to Dr. Goodlin, seniors may also be too thin because they are often alone and don't feel like eating. Increasing portion sizes of healthy foods, adding healthy snacks, eating cheese and yogurt, and drinking milk can help put on weight.

Dr. Goodlin stresses exercise for her patients. She notes that regular exercise is often not a part of senior citizens' approach to life. The emphasis on exercise really started with those who are now middle-aged. Many of Dr. Goodlin's patients do not realize that exercise can help them. An adequate amount of calcium is also important, according to Dr. Goodlin. Calcium supplements are best absorbed if taken with meals and spread out over the course of the day.

Dr. Goodlin would rather have her patients use exercise to address their physical discomfort and pain than take medications whenever possible. She has seen "huge differences" after her patients began exercising and eating properly.[43]

--- 7 ---

FRUITS AND VEGETABLES

"Live as our first parents did,
on fruits and on a little simple food."

—*Brigham Young*

People who eat five or six servings of fruits and vegetables a day may cut their risk of a stroke by almost a third, according to a recent Harvard study of health-care professionals. But one-half of Americans eat fewer than three servings.[44] Fruits and vegetables, along with grains, form the building blocks of the Word of Wisdom and are key to the Diet Solution. Because our health is influenced more and more by what we eat, it is not wise to skimp on these essential foods. Have them fresh, canned, or frozen. Eat a variety of them so that you benefit from all the nutrients they provide.

The great thing about fruits and vegetables for those trying to lose weight is that they provide fiber and many vitamins and minerals, but contain few calories, no cholesterol, and no fat (except avocados and coconut). The Food Guide Pyramid recommends two to four servings of fruit per day. If you are trying to lose weight, have the lowest number of servings. Don't worry about getting too much sugar from fruits. It is true that fruits contain sugar—fructose is the naturally occurring sugar in fruit. However fruits also contain vitamins A and C and potassium, as well as fiber. The sugars to watch out for are those in low-nutrient foods, such as candy and desserts. Dried fruits should be eaten in smaller amounts. They have more calories because there is less water in them, and the sugar is more concentrated. For example, one fresh apricot contains about 20 calories, but one-half cup dried apricots has about 150 calories. Apricots are rich in vitamin A, dried or fresh. Fruit juices have almost no fiber, so eat the whole fruit more often. Also, eat the skins of fruits for more fiber whenever possible.

Fruits are versatile. You can cook with them, bake with them, and have them in drinks and salads. You can even use pureed fruit in place of some of the fat in recipes. The fruit adds moisture, but because it does not melt like fat, the outcome is changed somewhat. Replace about one-fourth to one-half of the fat in your recipes and test the quality. You need to maintain at least one tablespoon of fat per cup of flour in the recipe. You will probably need to increase the baking time because the fruit will make the recipe extra moist.[45]

When you are fixing a dish, ask yourself how you could add fruit to it. Fortunately, children do not have the same aversion to fruit as they do to many vegetables, so provide them with a wide variety. Your family does not have to stick with the old standbys: apples, oranges, bananas, and grapes. Try mangoes for a change. They've got antioxidants, beta-carotene, vitamin C, and vitamin E. There are so many fruits to choose from that you could have something different every day of the week. The pioneers were limited by what they could grow themselves, the growing season, and the types of crops for their area. But we now have a worldwide market, which lets us have a variety of fruits and vegetables year round. It is still possible to grow and preserve your own fruits and vegetables, but that is not practical for many people. The next best alternative is to buy fruits and vegetables in season and eat or preserve them as quickly as possible. In-season produce is less expensive, better tasting, and more nutritious. Take advantage of farmers' markets in the summer. It would not be a bad idea to check with the produce person at your supermarket and find out when shipments come in. That way you can buy them at their freshest, rather than after the produce has sat around for several days.

The Food Guide Pyramid recommends three to five servings of vegetables each day. You do not have to stick to the lowest number of servings from the vegetable group because they have so little sugar and almost no fat. I have already talked about vegetables' cancer-fighting properties. Since so many varieties are available, why not introduce them to your family. You do not have to limit your diet to peas, corn, carrots, and potatoes. My son is not crazy about broccoli and cauliflower, but if I top them with a cheese sauce, he'll eat them right up. I've included my recipe in chapter 5. Stir-fry, pastas, casseroles, and soups are good ways to introduce many different types of vegetables. If you cook with celery you can cut back on your salt. Celery has a naturally salty flavor. Chapter 5 also includes a few recipes that call for zucchini and summer squash, which are both good vegetables to try out on your family. One thing to remember when cooking vegetables: The less they are cut up, the more nutrients are preserved. Cook them for the shortest amount of time and in the least amount of water. That way you will not lose all the water-soluble vitamins. Avoid peeling them when you can. Scrub the skins well and cook them or serve them with skins on. Mashed potatoes from new white potatoes, red potatoes, or Yukon Gold potatoes are great with the skins. Those packages of peeled and cut up carrots are handy, but if you wash carrots well with a vegetable brush and cut them yourself, you will have carrots with more fiber, and they are less expensive. Some diets you may have read say that you should not have white potatoes. Does that make sense? A diet with lots of white potatoes, especially if topped with sour cream and butter is not wise. But white potatoes in moderation are good for you. Sweet potatoes are not "better." Sweet potatoes supply vitamin A, while white potatoes, baked or otherwise, supply more vitamin C. Sweet potatoes have a little more fiber, but if the skin of the white potato is eaten, the fiber content turns out to be about the same. Eating a *variety* of fruits and vegetables is the best way to get all the benefits from these foods.

8

GRAINS

*"All grain is ordained for the use of man,
. . . to be the staff of life."*

—D&C 89:14

The Food Guide Pyramid recommends eating six to eleven servings from the grain group each day. This is easier than it sounds. If you are trying to lose weight, you'll want to keep to the lowest number of servings. Because each serving is only one-half cup, or one slice of bread, or one-half a bagel, the six servings can add up quickly. Try to have at least two or three of your servings each day from *whole-grain* foods. The whole grains provide the antioxidant vitamins A and E and selenium. They supply minerals such as zinc, copper, iron, and vitamin B6. And they are rich in complex carbohydrates and fiber, as well as being low in fat and cholesterol.[46]

Grains have sustained mankind for centuries, so it is incredible to read that many popular diets want you to avoid grains or drastically limit your consumption of them because they make you "fat." If grains are refined until there is little left but starch and if they are eaten to excess, then they may have that effect; however that is not what the Diet Solution or the Word of Wisdom are about. The importance of *whole* grains cannot be overstated. Refined grain products are OK in moderation. But it is so simple to upgrade the fiber content and nutritional value of food by adding whole-grain flour to white flour in recipes, or adding brown rice to white rice. After doing this, the switch to even more whole grains in your diet can be effortless and enjoyable.

WHEAT

Wheat is commonly used in the United States, but there are many other less familiar grains that are worth a try. Many of them have more protein than wheat. A protein content of 12 percent and above is the most desirable in hard wheat.[47] What makes wheat special is its versatility. It is the standard for bread making and cereals. If you have a wheat grinder, you can choose from different types of wheat. Lower-protein, soft wheat is used primarily for pastry flours and hard wheat for bread. Hard red wheat is the most common, but many bread makers say hard white wheat makes a milder tasting bread. If you like cooking with cracked wheat, just throw some wheat berries in the blender for a few seconds and you will have cracked wheat. Bulgur wheat is pre-cooked, dried cracked wheat. Because it is pre-cooked and can be stored for several months, it is an easy way to have wheat on hand for many dishes. A recipe for making bulgur and several other wheat recipes are included in chapter 5.

So, what are wheat bran and wheat germ? Wheat bran is the outer layer of the grain and provides B vitamins, fiber, and protein. The germ is the inside of the grain and also has B vitamins, protein, and vitamin E. The germ is what sprouts a new plant. Wheat germ has more protein; wheat bran has more fiber.[48] You do not need to buy special supplements or powders containing these foods. Just eat more whole wheat and you'll get both. Some members of my family are allergic to wheat. If you are like them, you can get your fiber, minerals, protein, and vitamins from other grains and foods. Wheat is not essential to your health.

Other Grains

• *Buckwheat* is high in protein and is used in many Russian and Eastern European dishes, such as kasha. The kernels are called groats. Buy the groats roasted and introduce them to your family in pancakes and hot cereal.

• *Triticale* is a cross between rye and wheat. It doesn't have enough gluten to bake with, but it is high in protein and can be used in casseroles and salads when the grain is cooked.

• *Quinoa* is a fast-cooking, high-protein South American grain. Try using it in place of rice or mixed with rice. Quinoa is becoming better known in the United States because it is so nutritious and easy to prepare.

• *Wild Rice* is actually the seed of a water grass. It has some protein and fiber and is great alone or mixed with rice or bulgur wheat.

• *Millet* is a tiny, round yellow grain that is not used much in the United States, except in birdseed. But it tastes good and is easy to toss into your bread dough, cooked cereal, or rice pilaf for added fiber. It cooks up fluffy or can be simmered with vegetables. To bring out millet's flavor you can dry roast it in a frying pan for about five minutes or until slightly browned. Your diet is not going to suffer if you never eat millet, but why not use a variety of grains when planning meals?

• *Barley* is one of my favorite grains. I love it in soups, stews, and casseroles. You can also try it as a stuffing for squash or cabbage. Most people buy pearl barley, which has the bran removed and cooks quickly. Whole-grain barley is also available for baking.

• *Rye* is most commonly used in Scandinavia and Germany. Rye does not have a lot of gluten so bread from rye flour will be heavy. You can add a little whole-grain rye to your wheat bread or other baked goods to get the rye flavor without the heaviness.

• *Corn* is a vegetable and a grain: a vegetable when it is eaten off the cob and a grain when it is dried and ground. Most wheat grinders can grind corn or you can buy it already ground. To get more fiber, have cornmeal muffins or cornbread sometimes instead of white rolls. Cornbread tastes especially good with stews, soups, and chili. A cup of unbuttered, lightly salted or no-salt popcorn makes a good snack. Hominy, or grits, is a southern United States dish made by drying the corn kernels and removing the hull. It is then soaked in liquid to soften the kernels, and cooked.

• *Oats*, a staple grain in Ireland and Scotland, is also popular in the United States, though more as a supplemental grain. For me, there is something very comforting about hot oatmeal cereal with raisins on a winter morning. Oats come in three forms: whole oats, with only the outer hull removed; scotch oats or steel-cut oats, which have been steamed and cut into pieces; and rolled oats that have been steamed and passed through rollers. Quick-cooking oats and instant oats are broken up even further. Whole oats are the most nutritious, but they take longer to prepare. Remember the oat bran craze of the 1980s? Oat bran was found to lower cholesterol under certain conditions. It seemed as though all of a sudden everything had oat bran in it. Oat bran is not a miracle food and it will not erase the effects of a high-fat diet, but the fiber in oat bran is good for you. Fiber is also in oatmeal, though not as much of it. The same kind of fiber can come from legumes, fruits, and vegetables. So again, there is no "magic bullet;" the best course is to eat a variety of healthy foods, and in most cases people will get the protective nutrition their bodies need.

• *Rice* is a staple food for most of the world's population. Brown rice is the whole, unpolished grain with only the inedible hull removed. Unfortunately, because of its stronger flavor and longer cooking time, it is not used as often as it could be in our diets. A good way to introduce it to your family would be to cook it separately and then mix it with cooked white rice. You can cook it in batches and freeze it, then add small amounts of it to white rice the last few minutes that the white rice is cooking.

There are three lengths of rice. Long grain rice is so called because its length is four to five times its width. Medium grain rice is about three times as long as its width. It is usually less expensive than long grain rice because it requires a shorter growing season, produces a higher yield, and is easier to mill. Short grain rice is only one and a half to two times as long as it is wide. There are also different types of rice. Regular milled white rice has the hull, germ, outer bran layers, and most of the inner bran removed. Parboiled or converted rice has been cooked before milling and treated to retain some of the nutrients that are in the whole grain. Enriched rice is a combination of fortified rice and regular milled rice. It is fortified with a coating of vitamins as well as the minerals thiamin, niacin, iron, and riboflavin. This coating does not dissolve with washing and cooking. What does dissolve are the B vitamins, which are added to rice in the form of powder. So you do not want to wash rice before cooking if it has been grown and milled in the United States. If you don't want gummy rice, do not stir the rice after it comes to a boil. If you do it will break up the grains.[49]

I hope I have encouraged you to add more whole grains to your diet. Grains freeze well, so cook up pots of several types and freeze. There are so many to try, and I think you will like the healthy change it can bring to the way you eat.

9

MEATS AND MEAT SUBSTITUTES

*"Fish is as healthy a food as we can eat, if we
except vegetables and fruit, and with them will
become a very wholesome diet."*

—*Brigham Young*

The apostle Paul said: "Now the Spirit speaketh expressly,
that in the latter times some shall depart from the faith,
giving heed to seducing spirits, and doctrines of devils; . . .
commanding to abstain from meats, which God hath created to be received with thanksgiving of them which
believe and know the truth. For every creature of God is
good, and nothing to be refused, if it be received with
thanksgiving" (1 Timothy 4:1–4).

From the Doctrine and Covenants we learn that "whoso
forbiddeth to abstain from meats, that man should not eat
the same, is not ordained of God; for, behold, the beasts of
the field and the fowls of the air, and that which cometh of
the earth, is ordained for the use of man for food and for
raiment, and that he might have in abundance" (49:18–19).

The Word of Wisdom says we are to eat meat sparingly.
The Food Guide Pyramid allows for two to three servings a
day from the Meat, Poultry, Fish, Dry Beans, Eggs, & Nuts
Group. A serving of meat is only two to three ounces, or

about the size of a deck of cards. With this information as our foundation, let's assume that you get all of your protein from meat—as opposed to the fish, dry beans, eggs, and nuts that are also a part of this group. If you eat only the minimum number of servings in the smallest serving sizes each day, your meat intake will be four to five ounces. Most likely, you eat more meat than this. Instead, simply follow the food pyramid's recommended number of servings, and you will already be eating healthier. Suppose that you also begin eating meats that are lower in fat and switch from a predominantly red-meat diet to a diet with more poultry and fish. This is even healthier. Now, if you were to go a step further and stop thinking of meat as a *necessary* part of your lunch and dinner each day, you would be well on your way to losing weight and taking better care of your body. There are many options besides meat that will give you the protein you need. I will get to them shortly. First, let me make it clear where I stand on meat. I do not think it is bad. I like meat. I like red meat. At a recent dinner party I was given the choice of prime rib, turkey, or salmon. I chose prime rib. Have I destroyed my health and disobeyed the Word of Wisdom? No. Before I made my choice I thought over what I had eaten the past week. I had had no red meat, several nights with no meat at all, and a couple of nights of fish for dinner. I felt perfectly comfortable with my decision and I enjoyed my meal. However, I did not eat the entire slab of prime rib that was heaped on my plate.

What I like about the Diet Solution is that it is all about knowing what your body needs and making choices. No one is telling you what you can and cannot eat or when you can eat. The Diet Solution is about "knowing correct principles and governing yourself." A diet is less restrictive this way and has a better chance of working over time because *you* are learning and making the decisions.

Americans get most of their protein from meat. Proteins are the building blocks of the body, and amino acids are the building blocks of protein. Proteins repair cells, build tissue, provide protection from disease, and ensure that certain chemical reactions occur in the body. There are nine essential amino acids that your body needs but cannot make itself. Meat—poultry, fish, and red meat—supplies all of these essential amino acids, so it is called a complete protein. Eggs, cheese, milk, and soybeans are also complete proteins. Other foods are considered incomplete proteins because they lack one or more of the nine essential amino acids. To make a complete protein you need to combine these foods with others. Grains combined with legumes make a complete protein. Rice and beans is an example of this combination. As long as your body gets all nine amino acids, it doesn't know or care whether they come from meat or a grain/legume combination. There is growing medical evidence that a diet with a lot of meat, especially red meat, can be bad for your health. The fat and cholesterol in meat can contribute to heart disease, cancer, and obesity. Scientists are now looking at a possible link between meat and non-Hodgkin's lymphoma, a cancer of the white blood cells. "Researchers from Harvard University reported that among more than 84,000 women, those who ate beef, pork or lamb as a main dish once a day had a higher risk of non-Hodgkin's lymphoma than those who ate meat less than once per week," according to an article in *The Dallas Morning News*.[50]

You *can* get the benefits of meat without eating too much of it. First, think of meat as a side dish and vegetables as your main dish, instead of the other way around. Second, prepare more casseroles, soups, stews, spaghetti sauce, salads, and stir-fry, where only small amounts of meat will be added. I recommend eating some meatless meals a few times a week. It can be a delicious and healthy break from the everyday meat routine. (Remember that one egg, a half-cup cooked beans, two tablespoons peanut butter, or a one-third cup nuts count as one ounce of lean meat or as one-third of a serving.) Try lentil or split pea soup with corn bread or whole-wheat bread; black beans and rice; chili and corn bread; corn tortillas and beans; macaroni and cheese casserole; or baked potatoes with low-fat yogurt topping. Use nuts and seeds more often. You do not need to use a lot. They are higher in fat than many other foods, so use them in moderation, and remember, the fat in nuts is unsaturated, so that's good. Buy nuts in bulk and store them in freezer bags in the freezer, ready to toss into casseroles, salads, and stir-fry. The recipe section in chapter 5 contains several ideas for low-meat or no-meat meals. Dry beans, dry peas, and lentils are nutritional small-food-budget bargains. They are inexpensive, and a little goes a long way. In addition, they contain B vitamins, calcium, and a lot of iron. Combined with a grain or a little meat, they also make a complete protein.

Soybeans are not used very often in America, but they are very nutritious. They contain one and one-half times more protein than other dry beans. (They also contain more fat, although it is the unsaturated kind.) Soybeans can be found in bulk in health food stores and some supermarkets. Several recent studies show that soy may help protect the body from some cancers, heart disease, bone loss, and prostate and menopause problems. Soybeans contain isoflavones, which are natural plant estrogens linked to lower rates of bone loss, fewer hot flashes and night sweats, and slower cancer cell growth in the prostate. Soy also helps lower cholesterol and makes arteries and blood tissues more elastic and reduces the risk of uterine cancer.[51] Not bad reasons to try some soy in your diet. I can get soymilk at my local supermarket and use it on cereal. It is not milky white like regular milk, but it tastes just fine.

10

FAT AND CHOLESTEROL

*"The people have laid the foundation of short life
through their diet, their rest, their labor, and their doing
this, that, and the other in a wrong manner, with
improper motives, and at improper times."*

—Brigham Young

How often have you heard the saying, "fat makes you fat?" It is true that each gram of fat provides nine calories, compared to four calories for proteins and carbohydrates. But that is not what makes us fat. *Too much* fat makes us fat, as does too much protein and too many carbohydrates. Some fat is good for you, especially the unsaturated type. Fat has a specific nutritional purpose and it is in our foods for a reason. Fat provides the body's most concentrated source of energy. It provides essential fatty acids, helps us absorb vitamins A, D, E, and K, provides insulation, makes food taste good, and gives us a full feeling. A diet with too little fat can turn out to be unhealthy, tasteless, and unsuccessful.

UNDERSTANDING THE LANGUAGE OF FAT

So, what is the skinny on fat? A fatty acid is a chain of carbon atoms. The body cannot make essential fatty acids itself; therefore they must come from the diet. There are three basic types of fats, all mixes of different fatty acids: *monounsaturated*, which is found in olive oil, peanut oil, and canola oil; *polyunsaturated*, which is found in corn oil, safflower oil (highest in polyunsaturated oil), soybean oil, and sesame seed oil; and *saturated*, which is found in meat, butter, dairy products, palm oil, coconut oil, and cocoa butter. (The term *saturated* refers to carbon atoms that are saturated with hydrogen.) Saturated fats are solid at room temperature and tend to increase cholesterol levels, as mentioned in chapter 4. Following is a chart showing the percentage of polyunsaturated, monounsaturated, and saturated fat in several different oils. Keep in mind when comparing butter and margarine, saturated and unsaturated fat, or polyunsaturated and monounsaturated fat that they still are 100 percent fat, though one may be healthier than another.

Fat Percentages

Type of Oil or Fat	Percent Poly-unsaturated	Percent Mono-unsaturated	Percent Saturated
Safflower oil	74	17	9
Sunflower oil	64	26	10
Corn oil	58	29	13
Average vegetable oil (soybean & cottonseed)	40	47	13
Peanut oil	30	51	19
Chicken fat (schmaltz)	26	45	29
Olive oil	9	77	14
Average vegetable shortening	20	48	32
Lard	12	48	40
Beef fat	4	48	48
Butter	4	35	61
Palm oil	2	17	82
Coconut oil	2	12	86

Source: Utah State University Extension

The term *hydrogenated fat* refers to a liquid fat that has been changed to solid form by adding hydrogen, as in shortening and some margarines. Another term often associated with fat is *omega-3 fatty acid*. It is a polyunsaturated fat found in abundance in fish, especially tuna and salmon, and has been shown in some research to help prevent heart disease. The term *triglyceride* is a fancy way of saying fat— most of the fat we consume and store in the body is made up of triglycerides. A triglyceride is a glycerol molecule to which three fatty acids are linked. I do not want this to start sounding like a chemistry lesson, but a few basics will help you understand the lingo when these and other terms are thrown around. *Lipid* is the scientific term for fat and fat-like substances, such as cholesterol. That is where the word *liposuction* comes from. Lipids are not soluble in water. To get through the body in the bloodstream they are coated with a protein substance and referred to as *lipoproteins*. This is where HDL and LDL, referring to "good" and "bad" cholesterol, come in. The liver produces most of the cholesterol your body needs. But because animals produce cholesterol, you are taking in more cholesterol when you eat animal products. (Foods from plants do not contain cholesterol.)[52]

Too much cholesterol in the bloodstream can cause fatty deposits to form in the arteries, which then slow the flow of blood through the body, resulting in a heart attack or stroke. High-density lipoproteins (HDL), which have a higher percent of protein and less cholesterol and triglycerides, pick up cholesterol from the body and take it to the liver where the body disposes of it. Low-density lipoproteins (LDL), which have a higher percentage of cholesterol and triglycerides and a lower percentage of protein, work in reverse, delivering cholesterol to the cells.[53] You want to have higher HDL readings and lower LDL readings when your cholesterol is checked. HDL can be raised and LDL lowered by losing weight, exercising, eating less saturated fat, and eating more fiber. Total blood cholesterol should be less than

200 mg, LDL should be less than 130 mg, and HDL should be at least, or more than 35 mg.[54]

A product that says it is cholesterol free is not necessarily fat free, so check the labels. Following are charts from the U.S. Department of Agriculture showing the grams of fat in many of the foods in the Food Guide Pyramid.

Bread, Cereal, Rice, and Pasta Group

Eat 6 to 11 servings daily	Servings	Grams of Fat
Bread, 1 slice	1	1
Hamburger roll, bagel, English muffin, 1	2	2
Tortilla, 1	1	3
Rice, pasta, cooked, $^1/_2$ cup	1	Trace
Plain crackers, small, 3–4	1	3
Breakfast cereal, 1 oz.	1	*
Pancakes, 4" diameter, 2	2	3
Croissant, 1 large (2 oz.)	2	12
Doughnut, 1 medium (2 oz.)	2	11
Danish, 1 medium (2 oz.)	2	13
Cake, frosted, $^1/_{16}$ average	1	13
Cookies, 2 medium	1	4
Pie, fruit, 2-crust, $^1/_6$ 8" pie	2	19

*Check product label.

Vegetable Group

Eat 3 to 5 servings daily	Servings	Grams of Fat
Vegetables, cooked, $^1/_2$ cup	1	Trace
Vegetables, leafy, raw, 1 cup	1	Trace
Vegetables, nonleafy, raw, chopped, $^1/_2$ cup	1	Trace
Potatoes, scalloped, $^1/_2$ cup	1	4
Potato salad, $^1/_2$ cup	1	8
French fries, 10	1	8

Fruit Group

Eat 2 to 4 servings daily	Servings	Grams of Fat
Whole fruit: medium apple, orange, banana	1	Trace
Fruit, raw or canned, $^1/_2$ cup	1	Trace
Fruit juice, unsweetened, $^3/_4$ cup	1	Trace
Avocado, $^1/_4$ whole	1	9

Milk, Yogurt, and Cheese Group

Eat 2 to 3 servings daily	Servings	Grams of Fat
Skim milk, 1 cup	1	Trace
Nonfat yogurt, plain, 8 oz.	1	Trace
Low-fat milk, 2 percent, 1 cup	1	5
Whole milk, 1 cup	1	8
Chocolate milk, 2 percent, 1 cup	1	5
Low-fat yogurt, plain, 8 oz.	1	4
Low-fat yogurt, fruit, 8 oz.	1	3
Natural cheddar cheese, $1^1/_2$ oz.	1	14
Process cheese, 2 oz.	1	18
Mozzarella, part skim, $1^1/_2$ oz.	1	7
Ricotta, part skim, $^1/_2$ cup	1	10
Cottage cheese, 4 percent fat, $^1/_2$ cup	$^1/_4$	5
Ice cream, $^1/_2$ cup	$^1/_3$	7
Ice milk, $^1/_2$ cup	$^1/_3$	3
Frozen yogurt, $^1/_2$ cup	$^1/_2$	2

Meat, Poultry, Fish, Dry Beans, Eggs, and Nuts Group

Eat 5 to 7 oz. daily	Servings	Grams of Fat
Lean meat, poultry, fish, cooked	3 oz.*	6
Ground beef, lean, cooked	3 oz.*	16
Chicken, with skin, fried	3 oz.*	13
Bologna, 2 slices	1 oz.*	16
Egg, 1	1 oz.*	5
Dry beans and peas, cooked, ¹/₂ cup	1 oz.*	Trace
Peanut butter, 2 tbsp.	1 oz.*	16
Nuts, ¹/₃ cup	1 oz.*	22

*Ounces of meat these items count as

Fats, Oils, and Sweets

Use sparingly	Servings	Grams of fat
Butter, margarine, 1 tsp.	-	4
Mayonnaise, 1 tbsp.	-	11
Salad dressing, 1 tbsp.	-	7
Reduced calorie salad dressing, 1 tbsp.	-	*
Sour cream, 2 tbsp.	-	6
Cream cheese, 1 oz.	-	10
Sugar, jam, jelly, 1 tsp.	-	0
Cola, 12 fl. oz.	-	0
Fruit drink, ade, 12 fl. oz.	-	0
Chocolate bar, 1 oz.	-	9
Sherbet, ¹/₂ cup	-	2
Fruit sorbet, ¹/₂ cup	-	0
Gelatin dessert, ¹/₂ cup	-	0

* Check product label

Brigham Young University's "Y-B-Fit" wellness program provides its clients with a list of ways to decrease the fat in your diet. Here are some of their ideas:

• Cook with non-fat powdered milk.

• Sop up extra fat from cooked bacon or sausage by pressing between paper towels.

• Drink skim milk, which has basically no fat and only 5 mg cholesterol, compared to whole milk with 8.5 grams of fat and 34 mg of cholesterol. (Children between one and three years of age should drink whole milk.)

• Use low-fat yogurt on potatoes, and in dips, salad dressings, and recipes that call for sour cream or mayonnaise. A cup of low-fat yogurt has about 3.5 grams of fat, 11 mg of cholesterol, and 150 calories. Sour cream has 47.5 grams fat, 152 mg cholesterol, and 475 calories. Mayonnaise has 176.5 grams of fat, 155 mg cholesterol, and 1,600 calories.

• Prepare stews, soups, or other dishes in which fat cooks into the liquid a day ahead of time and then refrigerate. It is easy to remove the hardened fat before re-heating.

• Chill canned foods before opening, and then remove the hardened fat.

• Add a few ice cubes to meat drippings when making gravy. The fat will cling to the ice cubes. Discard and voila, low-fat gravy.

• Puree cooked vegetables in a blender. Use the puree to thicken soups and stews instead of fats or starches.

• Be careful at salad bars. Adding chopped ham, cheddar cheese, marinated vegetables, and dressing may add more than 30 grams of fat.

---11---

SUGAR AND SALT

*"Yea, all things which come of the earth, in the
season thereof, are made for the benefit and the use of
man. . . . And it pleaseth God that he hath given all
these things unto man; for unto this end were they
made to be used, with judgment, not to excess."*

—*D&C 59:18–20*

Sugar does not make you fat—it is a simple carbohydrate that contains about 16 calories per teaspoon. The problem with sugar—besides contributing to tooth decay, of course—is that it supplies no nutrients and may replace healthy food. How often have you been in a rush and grabbed a candy bar instead of having a nutritious meal just because it was easy and gave you a jolt of energy? Choosing foods high in complex carbohydrates—such as grains, vegetables, and fruits—instead of foods made up of the simple carbohydrates found in sugars will supply nutrients and fiber along with added energy. Be careful though, if you eat more calories than your body needs, some of the natural sugar found in fruits and vegetables can be converted and stored as fat.

Most of the sugars with which we are familiar contain the same number of calories per teaspoon. Brown sugar—

which is either regular sugar that has been dyed with molasses or sugar that has come from sugar canes naturally rich in brown syrup—contains 15 calories per teaspoon. Honey has a few more calories than sugar, but you are likely to use less of it because it is sweeter than sugar. One note about honey: Some honey producers claim honey is an antioxidant. But nutritionists say that honey is no better for you than regular sugar; the amount of nutrients in honey is too small to make a big difference. Honey should never be given to infants because it can contain harmful botulism spores, which are potentially fatal in children this age.

While many people are concerned about blood sugar levels, insulin resistance, and other health issues related to sugar, this book covers only the basics of nutrition and sugar. Your blood sugar level and what it means for your health is best discussed with your doctor.

Read food labels to know how much added sugar you are getting and whether the food has plenty of nutrients to offer in addition to the sugar. A *tablespoon* of sugar and a small orange have about the same amount of calories, but what a difference in nutrition! With sugar, as with most things, moderation is the key. Unfortunately for some, moderation is really hard when it comes to sweets. To begin cutting down, try sharing your desserts with a spouse, friend, or one of your children. What can help you even more, however, is learning how to practice moderation in all things. Section 3, which discusses spiritual nourishment, will address this.

Following is a chart from the U.S. Department of Agriculture that shows where added sugars come from in various food groups.

Sugar in Food Groups

Bread, Cereal, Rice, and Pasta Group	Added Sugars (teaspoons)
Bread, 1 slice	0
Muffin, 1 medium	1
Cookies, 2 medium	1
Danish pastry, 1 medium	1
Doughnut, 1 medium	2
Ready-to-eat cereal, sweetened, 1 oz.	*
Pound cake, no-fat, 1 oz.	2
Angelfood cake, $1/12$ tube cake	5
Cake, frosted, $1/16$ average	6
Pie, fruit, 2 crust, $1/6$ 8" pie	6

Fruit Group	
Fruit, canned in juice, $1/2$ cup	0
Fruit, canned in light syrup, $1/2$ cup	2
Fruit, canned in heavy syrup, $1/2$ cup	4

Milk, Yogurt, and Cheese Group	
Milk, plain, 1 cup	0
Chocolate milk, 2 percent, 1 cup	3
Low-fat yogurt, plain, 8 oz.	0
Low-fat yogurt, flavored, 8 oz.	5
Low-fat yogurt, fruit, 8 oz.	7
Ice cream, ice milk, or frozen yogurt, $1/2$ cup	3
Chocolate shake, 10 fl. oz.	9

Other	Added Sugars (teaspoons)
Sugar, jam, or jelly, 1 tsp.	1
Syrup or honey, 1 tbsp.	3
Chocolate bar, 1 oz.	3
Fruit sorbet, $^1/_2$ cup	3
Gelatin dessert, $^1/_2$ cup	4
Sherbet, $^1/_2$ cup	5
Cola, 12 fl. oz.	9
Fruit drink, ade, 12 fl. oz.	12

Check product label

SODIUM

In most people, the body rids itself of the sodium it does not need. But for the overweight and inactive and those who smoke and drink, too much sodium can pose a hazard, especially if they tend to have high blood pressure. With so much focus on the negative aspects of sodium, it's easy to forget that the right amount of sodium is actually good for us. Sodium and other minerals, such as potassium, are called electrolytes. They perform essential functions, such as maintaining proper fluid balance, transmitting nerve impulses, and making muscles, including the heart, contract. With sodium intake, moderation is again the key, even if you are healthy. You should not have more than 2,000 to 3,000 mg of sodium a day. This is a little less than one teaspoon. Most of the sodium we get comes from processed and prepared foods, not from what we add at the dinner table. You may not think you are getting too much sodium, but you could be surprised. Check the nutrition labels on the foods you buy and try not to buy a lot of already prepared food. Following is a chart from the U.S. Department of Agriculture that shows how much sodium is found in some common foods.

Sodium in Food Groups

Bread, Cereal, Rice, and Pasta Group	Sodium, mg
Cooked cereal, rice, pasta, unsalted, $^1/_2$ cup	Trace
Ready-to-eat cereal, 1 oz.	100–360
Bread, 1 slice	110–175
Popcorn, salted, 1 oz.	100–420
Pretzels, salted, 1 oz.	130–880

Vegetable Group	
Vegetables, fresh or frozen, cooked without salt, $^1/_2$ cup	Less than 70
Vegetables, canned or frozen with sauce, $^1/_2$ cup	140–460
Tomato juice, canned, $^3/_4$ cup	660
Vegetable soup, canned, 1 cup	820

Fruit Group	
Fruit, fresh, frozen, canned, $^1/_2$ cup	Trace

Milk, Yogurt, and Cheese Group	
Milk, 1 cup	120
Yogurt, 8 oz.	160
Natural cheeses, $1^1/_2$ oz.	110–450
Process cheeses, 2 oz.	800

Meat, Poultry, Fish, Dry Beans, Eggs, and Nuts Group	
Fresh meat, poultry, fish, 3 oz.	Less than 90
Tuna, canned, water pack, 3 oz.	300
Bologna, 2 oz.	580
Ham, lean, roasted, 3 oz.	1,020
Peanuts, roasted in oil, salted, 1 oz.	120

Other	Sodium, mg
Salad dressing, 1 tbsp.	75–220
Ketchup, mustard, steak sauce, 1 tbsp.	130–230
Soy sauce, 1 tbsp.	1,030
Salt, 1 tsp.	2,325
Dill pickle, 1 medium	930

SECTION TWO

Exercise

12

AEROBIC EXERCISE

*"As for health, it is far healthier to walk than to ride,
and better every way for the people."*

—*Brigham Young*

The word *aerobic* means "with oxygen." An aerobic exercise is one in which the large muscles of your body (arms and legs) move in continuous, rhythmical motion, raising your heart rate to between 60 percent and 90 percent of maximum. "The maximum heart rate is the maximum number of beats per minute that the heart can attain. It is dependent on age and can be estimated by subtracting one's age from 220."[55] For example, if you are 45 years old, you have a maximum heart rate of 175 beats per minute. You should exercise at a pace that keeps your heart rate between 105 and 157 beats per minute. This is your aerobic training range. In this range, carbohydrates *and fats* are burned, and oxygen reaches your muscles, where it is converted into muscular energy. If, when you are exercising, you are breathing hard but still can carry on a conversation you know you are in your aerobic range. If you are out of breath and cannot talk, your exercise will not be as effective and you may experience more muscle soreness. In addition you will not be able to keep up this pace long enough to burn fat as an energy source.

You will need to be able to find your pulse to determine your heart rate and learn to stay within your aerobic range. During your exercise session, stop once in a while for just a bit and check your pulse. Do it immediately because the pulse will drop rapidly. Starting from zero, count the number of heartbeats for ten seconds, then multiply that number by six to find your heart rate per minute. My pulse is so faint that I cannot find it reliably, so I purchased a monitor from a sporting goods shop. If you are interested in one, get the type that consists of a wristwatch and a strap that goes around the chest. The kind that measures heart rate by a device on the finger is not as good. Most important, *get your doctor's OK before you start an exercise program.*

Running, jogging, swimming, skating, bicycling, rowing, cross country skiing, and jump roping are all examples of aerobic activities. Even gardening can be an aerobic activity. Most fitness experts recommend getting twenty to sixty minutes of continuous aerobic activity, three to five days per week. If you have not exercised for quite a while, start off slowly. It will take you longer to get fit, but do not get discouraged. Begin at three days per week and twenty minutes per day. If even this seems too difficult, try ten minutes, twice per day, then work your way up.

For those who are not new to exercise and want to lose weight, exercise five days a week when possible. Later you can drop to three times a week to maintain the weight. The duration of each session depends on the type of activity. A lower intensity activity (meaning at the lower end of the heart rate range) should be performed for a longer period of time. Taking time in the day to exercise for the *minimum* of twenty minutes is doable for just about anyone. The more fit you become, the less tired you will be in general and when exercising. You will also be strengthening your heart muscle, enabling it to pump more blood with each beat.

This in turn makes it possible for your heart to beat less often to supply the same amount of blood to the body. And to put it simply, this means your heart will last longer.

It is better to eat *after* you exercise, because your metabolism is then elevated. But if you eat first, wait thirty to forty-five minutes to allow your food to settle.

WARM UP

Always warm up and stretch before you begin your aerobic exercise. Then, after your exercise, cool down and stretch again. You do not want to stop abruptly and go sit or lie down. Warm up or cool down by slowing your walk for about five to ten minutes. Stretch your **hamstrings** by standing on one leg and propping the other leg parallel to the ground on a table. Bend over and slide your hands toward the propped-up ankle as far as they will go, but do not bounce. Repeat with the other leg. The **quadriceps** stretch is done by putting your left hand on a wall or tree to steady yourself, then reaching behind your back with the right hand and grabbing the ankle of the right leg. Pull it up toward your bottom until you feel the stretch in the front of your thigh. Repeat on the opposite side. Stretch the **Achilles tendon** and **calf muscles** by placing both hands against a wall or tree. Place one foot way behind you. Keep the rear leg straight with its heel on the ground and lean in toward the wall or tree. Repeat with the other leg.

GETTING STARTED

One of the easiest and least expensive ways to get aerobic exercise is walking. I try to walk forty-five minutes a day, five days a week. Sometimes I do more if I can, and sometimes I have to do less. Once in a while I like to in-line skate instead. And in the winter I occasionally cross-country ski. But basically I am a walker. When the weather is bad, I get out an exercise video and a step. A treadmill is great to have, but not necessary. Shawn Fluharty, my exercise adviser for this book, told me the most reasonable and best training range for weight loss is 65 to 85 percent of my maximum heart rate, for an accumulation of thirty to sixty minutes per day, four to five times a week. I like to get the workout in all at once, but you can break it up during the day. You can even do your aerobics in the evening. Sometimes I do twenty minutes before I go to bed. It does not keep me awake afterwards. In fact, it helps me sleep, provided I cool down and stretch when I am finished.

Here is a good way to find out how your aerobic fitness is progressing: Get in your car and measure off a three-mile distance. Then walk it, keeping within your aerobic range, and see how long it takes. About every four or five weeks, walk that route again and see if you can finish it faster each time, still staying within your range. *The more fit you become, the more you should vary your exercise routine.* Your body will soon get used to the same old walk and the benefits from it will begin to diminish. The body gets conditioned to certain intensities, thus necessitating an increase. To do this, just change the exercise a bit. For example, take a new route that includes hills; carry hand weights (even soup cans will do); raise your arms over your head or at heart level while you are walking (if you have heart problems, you should not raise your arms above your head); walk on an unpaved road instead of a paved road; or put on a weighted backpack. Each of these things will increase the intensity of your exercise and may even get you off one of those discouraging weight plateaus. If you have a lot of weight to lose, you will lose with less effort at first. Then, as the weight starts coming off, you will have to increase the intensity of your workout to keep losing weight. If you are using a treadmill, put it on an incline. If you are using a step, increase the height or go for a more difficult routine. You can intersperse a walk with periods of more speed. For example, walk three blocks, then jog one block. When you feel ready, walk two blocks and jog one block. After a few more days, walk one block and jog one block. Just make sure you are monitoring your heart rate to stay within the aerobic zone. Initially you may vary your exercise weekly; later, try for daily or twice weekly. Call your local parks and recreation department for some good hiking and nature trails to get a change of scene for your mind and your muscles.

When you walk, be sure it is a fitness walk, not a stroll. In a fitness walk you step from the hip, using the whole leg with a full stride. Do not lean forward when walking, lean back slightly. (I tried this and noticed a big change. I could feel the leg working harder and stretching further. Plus, by leaning back slightly you get more resistance.) Feel the weight on your heel first. Keep the upper body firm, not loose, and tilt your pelvis up. When you want to swing your arms, swing them from the shoulder with your elbows bent at a 90-degree angle. Breathe deeply when you exercise. Drink plenty of water before, during, and after you exercise. You will not need a sports drink to replace electrolytes because you probably will not be exercising long enough to need electrolyte replacement.

EXERCISE FOR THE WHOLE FAMILY

Make exercise part of your family's time together. *Always wear protective gear:* helmet, kneepads, and so on, depending on the exercise. Plan activities like you plan your meals. You may want to make up a calendar each month with family events and exercise days on it. You could even have an exercise theme for each month, perhaps centering on an Olympic event. You may even want to make up your own Olympics. Swimming is a good family activity, as are walks, bicycle rides, and hikes. As a game, time your family walks and try to beat your previous time. Another idea is to make an activity box filled with descriptions of different types of exercise and sports. Once a week someone draws an activity from the box, and that becomes the family's exercise for the week. Participate as a family in the Presidential Sports Award program, which is sponsored by the President's Council on Physical Fitness and Sports and the Amateur Athletic Union. Anyone over six years of age is eligible. To find out more you can write to the Presidential Sports Award, c/o Walt Disney World Resort, P.O. Box 10,000, Lake Buena Vista, FL 32839–1000. Tel. 407–934–7200. Fax 407–934–7242. Have fun!

13

STRENGTH TRAINING AND TONING

"My mind becomes tired, and perhaps some of yours do.
If so, go and exercise your bodies."

—*Brigham Young*

Before you start strength training and toning, get the OK from your doctor. Show the doctor the exercises you plan to do. I have chosen exercises here that people of all ages can do. Start the strength training and toning portion of your exercise routine by taking your measurements: chest, waist, forearms, hips, and thighs. Note where on your arms, stomach, and so on, you took the measurements so that you can take them in the same place each time—about once a month. The waist measurement should be taken at the navel level. Measure your hips at the widest part. You may see a loss in your size before you see a big loss in pounds. This can be particularly true when you reach one of those weight plateaus. Also, remember there is no ideal weight. Your best weight depends on your percentage of body fat and how healthy you are. For most women, an acceptable body fat percentage is between 20 and 30 percent; for men it is 12 to 20 percent. Several different methods can be used to test body fat percentage. The most accurate but also the most expensive method is hydrostatic weighing, in which you are dunked in a tank of water and weighed. Your weight underwater is then compared with your weight on land. Another method is a skin fold caliper test. In this test, you are pinched at different points on your body with something that looks like a pair of pliers. This measures the thickness of the fat layer under your skin. It is fast and relatively inexpensive. Health clinics and wellness centers at universities or hospitals can perform this test. Some health clubs also offer the service. If you do not want to bother with these tests, the best way to know if you are losing fat is to take your waist, hip, and chest measurements periodically.

A few facts of life before we start: First, fat does not change into muscle. Fat and muscle are completely different substances. Muscle, however, burns more calories than fat. Second, "Use it or lose it." No matter how long you keep with a strength-training program, once you give it up for a few months you will eventually lose the muscle mass and be back where you started. However, the good news is that if you start up your strength training again, it will not take as long to get in shape as it did the first time. Third, you can tone, firm, and build muscles in any area of your body, but you cannot earmark a specific part of your body for fat loss. This is most unfortunate, since many of us women would like to keep a little padding in some places and not in others.

Strength training has many benefits, especially as we age. We will be less injury prone, we will lose less muscle mass, we will be stronger longer, we can be independent longer, our bad cholesterol will be lower, and our good cholesterol will be higher, and we will ward off osteoporosis because our bones will be denser.

Dieting without strength training can make us shed fat *and* muscle, changing us from flabby and weak to thin and weak. So begin now with the following strength training exercises. They require several sets of dumbbells: three-pound, five-pound, and eight-pound. You can start off using soup cans. Get heavier weights later if you need them. The exercises also require some surgical tubing or exercise bands. You can do just the tubing or band exercises, instead of those using weights if you want. But the more variety in your exercises the better. I bought my surgical tubing and exercise bands at a medical supply store. They are not expensive. I prefer using the bands because they are wider and more comfortable. Buy bands in different tensions. I bought a medium-tension band and a harder-tension band. Light-tension bands are also available. You can change the tension of bands and surgical tubing by making them shorter or longer. Buy two two-foot lengths of tubing. A couple of other useful and inexpensive pieces of exercise equipment include a large exercise ball which you can get from a sporting goods store and a child's ball, about six inches in diameter. For a change from the exercises in this book, you can rent or buy your own strength training videos. Rent some first to try them out. You cannot stick to just one video however, because your muscles adapt to the same exercises after a few weeks and you will not get results. Your muscles *need* to be challenged.

The strength and toning exercises listed here can be done twice a week, but not more than three times a week if you are doing all of them— upper body and lower body—at once. Your muscles need off days to repair themselves. This is true for all but the stomach exercises and the thigh exercises that are done without bands or weights. These can be done daily, if you want. You also have the choice of alternating days by doing upper body exercises one day and lower body exercises the next. Choose whichever system works best for your schedule. I prefer doing them all at once, then skipping a day or two.

Most of the exercises here consist of two to three sets of eight to twelve repetitions (reps) each. When you are no longer fatigued at twelve reps you can add more sets or do more reps. When using weights, you can increase the weight whenever you feel ready, and continue to do so, until you reach the limit that you can lift. Lifting heavier weights in fewer repetitions is called the overload principle and can really change your body composition from more fat to more muscle although you won't look like a body builder. A note about protein: Your diet has more than enough protein for muscle building, without having to use supplements. As you exercise you will be building lean muscle mass. The larger the lean muscle mass, the more calories your body burns. "Pound for pound, muscle burns 40 to 50 more calories a day than fat burns. So putting on just three pounds of muscle will consume an extra 120 to 150 extra calories every 24 hours, even while you sleep."[56] Sound good? Now, let's get started and remember to have your water on hand.

STRENGTH AND TONING EXERCISES

Do not do all of the exercises at once—there are enough so you can switch them around every week or so. Pick upper body, stomach, and lower body exercises and do a total of eight sets (from eight to fifteen reps per set) each session. If you cannot do eight reps, the weight you are using is too heavy. The last rep should be difficult. Keep in mind that you should not work more than two or three muscle groups per exercise session. Make each movement slow and controlled. Exhale on the exertion stage of the exercise and inhale on the recovery stage. Keep the stomach muscles firm. Any of the band exercises can be done with tubing instead.

Upper Body Exercises

Chest Press with Band

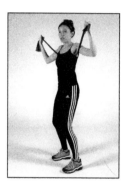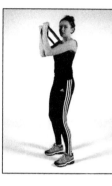

1. Place the band around the upper back and under the armpits.

2. Hold on to the ends of the band and adjust the length by wrapping it around your hands to get the desired tension. Keep the elbows bent with the hands at forehead height and press the elbows into the center of the body.

3. Return to the starting position. Do eight to ten, rest, and repeat if you can.

Extended Chest Press with Band

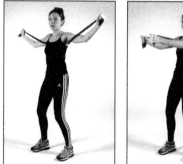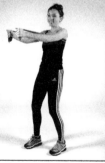

1. Place the band around the upper back and under the armpits.

2. Keep your arms straight, and move your hands towards each other so they meet in front of your chest, arms extended. Do eight to ten, rest, and try to repeat.

Lat Pull Downs

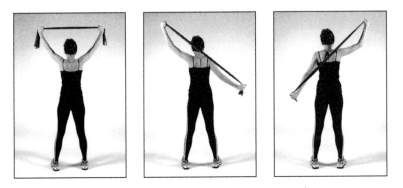

1. Hold the ends of the band in each hand, over your head. Keep as strong a tension as you can.

2. Lower first one arm and then the other behind your head, elbows slightly bent until you have stretched as far down as possible.

3. Slowly raise again each arm back over your head. Do ten to fifteen reps, rest, and repeat.

Seated Row

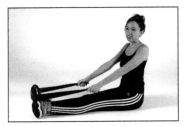 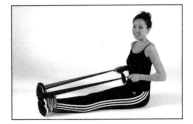

1. Sit up with your legs extended in front of you.

2. Hook the band around the soles of your feet, holding each end with your hands at knee level.

3. Pull the ends of the band towards you with your elbows close to your sides and your back straight.

4. Slowly return to starting position. Do fifteen reps, rest, and repeat.

Shoulder Press

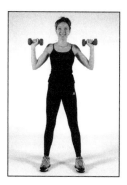 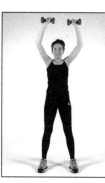

1. Standing with feet shoulder-width apart and knees slightly bent, take dumbbells (start out light if you need to) with both hands.

2. With palms facing forward and elbows all the way down, lift the dumbbells slowly straight up over your head, pausing at ear level.

3. Return slowly. Do fifteen times and repeat.

Biceps Curls

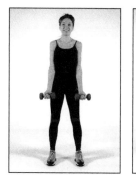 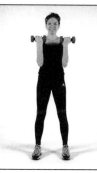

1. In standing position, hold dumbbells at sides with palms facing forward.

2. Slowly curl up dumbbells to chest level.

3. Return to starting position, slow and controlled. Do fifteen reps and repeat if you can.

Chest Fly

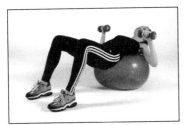 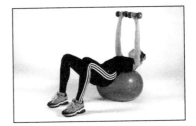

1. Lie on back on ball to get the full range of motion with your arms. Have knees bent, feet flat on floor.

2. Take dumbbells and extend arms, elbows slightly bent.

3. Move arms overhead until hands are two inches apart.

4. Lower arms with elbows bent until upper arms are as close to the floor as possible. Do fifteen times and repeat if possible.

Modified Push-up

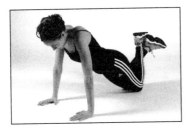 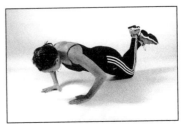

1. Get on hands and knees, with hands shoulder-width apart, fingers pointing forward.

2. Lift calves off the floor and cross ankles.

3. Lower body toward floor until elbows are at a 90-degree angle. Keep back flat.

4. Push straight up. Repeat as many times as you can. The first thing to touch the floor should be your nose, not your thighs. You should be on the upper part of the knee, not the kneecap. If these are too difficult, you can try doing standing push-ups against a wall at first.

Chair Dip

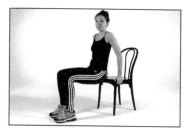

1. Sit on the edge of a chair with legs extended and hands holding onto the seat alongside your hips.

2. Keeping your arms straight, slide your bottom off the chair and bend the knees slightly so your feet are flat on the floor.

3. Lower your body, bending the elbows until the upper arms are parallel to the floor.

4. Pause and slowly push yourself back up. These are tough. Do as many as you can, working up to ten times. Remember to keep your body close to the chair.

Triceps Extension

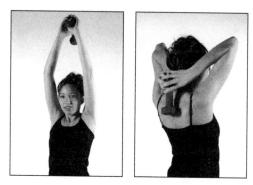

1. Stand with back straight and knees slightly bent.

2. Hold a three- to five-pound dumbbell with both hands and raise it over your head, elbows in close.

3. Relax, and let the weight dangle towards the floor behind your head.

4. Keeping arms close to your head and bending the elbows, lower the weight behind your head as far as you can.

5. Pause, and lift the weight slowly back up. Repeat as many times as you can, working up to twenty reps. Be sure to keep your elbows close to your ears at all times.

Triceps Kickback

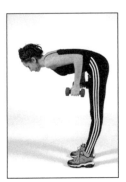 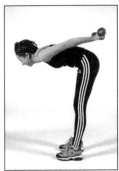

1. Bend at the waist, with your elbows bent 90 degrees.

2. Hold a three- to five-pound dumbbell in each hand. Keep shoulders relaxed and elbows close to your body.

3. Point your palms inward, your hands in front of your hips.

4. From the elbow, move your arms straight behind you and rotate your palms so they face upward. Keep upper arms still. Repeat up to ten times.

Lying French Press

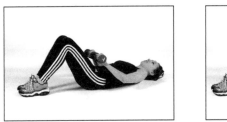 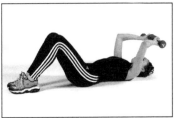

1. Lie on your back with knees bent and feet flat on floor. If you have an aerobic's step, lie on it so your bottom is just at the end.

2. With palms facing the floor, take a bar or dumbbells (keeping them even) and raise them until your hands are over your shoulders, elbows relaxed.

3. Keeping your upper arms still, slowly lower the bar or dumbbells toward your head, until arms are at right angles.

4. Return until your hands are over your shoulders again. Repeat ten to fifteen times. Do two more sets.

Stretches

Do this after each exercise session.

1. Stand tall and roll your shoulders back several times.

2. Then roll them forward several times.

3. Next, take your left arm straight across your upper body and push it toward your chest with your right arm.

4. Repeat with the other arm.

Abdominals

Abdominals can be done every day. When doing them, always exhale as you sit up and inhale as you lie back down.

Crunch

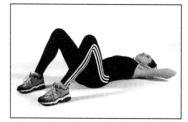 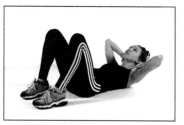

Do up to three sets of eight to twelve reps.

1. Lie on a mat or towel, eyes facing the ceiling, fingertips behind your head, elbows out. Have knees bent, feet flat on the floor.

2. Using your stomach muscles (abs), lift your head and shoulder blades off the floor, but keep your lower back on the floor. Do not pull up with your head. Take three seconds to curl up.

3. Hold for three seconds.

4. Take three seconds to curl back down.

Oblique Crunch

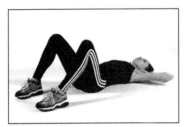 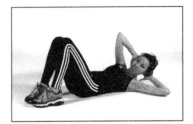

1. Lie on a mat or towel, eyes facing the ceiling, hands lightly touching the sides of your head.

2. As you slowly curl your head and shoulders off the floor, twist your upper body so your right elbow is pointing toward your left knee. Lie back down, then curl your head and shoulders off the floor again, twisting to the right so your left elbow is pointing toward your right knee. Alternate from side to side as many times as you can.

Reverse Crunch

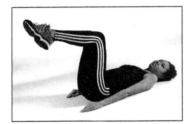 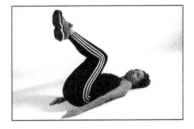

1. Lie flat on your back, arms straight down at the sides.

2. Lift your knees so your shins are parallel to the floor.

3. Slowly curl knees toward the chest, pressing your lower back into the floor.

4. Slowly lower back until shins are parallel to the floor again. Repeat for one minute.

Stretches

1. Lie on your back, legs out straight, and feet pointed. Arms should be straight behind you, close to your head.

2. Simultaneously stretch your legs toward your toes and your arms toward your fingertips. Hold for 30 seconds.

3. Turn over so you are face down on the floor and your arms are extended in front of you.

4. Lift your right leg and your left arm.

5. Hold the stretch, then lower.

6. Switch sides and repeat.

Lower Body Exercises

Just a few notes before you get started. Do not do pliés, squats, or lunges if you have knee problems. Pay attention to your breathing: Exhale on exertion, inhale on recovery. Move slowly and deliberately. Keep stomach tight. Any of the band exercises can be done with tubing instead.

Pliés

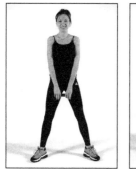 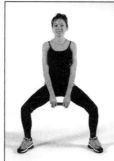

1. Stand with feet a little more than shoulder-width apart, toes pointing out, and knees slightly bent.

2. Hold a dumbbell with both hands between legs.

3. Bend your knees until they are at a 90-degree angle. Keep your back straight; knees should not go beyond toes—you should be able to see your toes, otherwise the position is wrong.

4. Return to starting position. Try this exercise first without weight, holding onto a chair for balance.

Squat

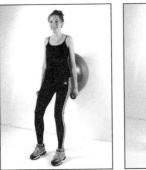 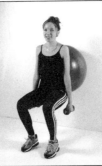

It is important in this exercise to have proper form, which is why we are using the large exercise ball. It is a great exercise. In fact, when you do not have time for several lower-body exercises, do this one instead. You can do it with or without the weights.

1. Start in a standing position, feet shoulder-width apart. Your weight should be on your heels and the ball should be between the wall and your back.

2. Hold the dumbbells in each hand at mid-thigh; do not push back into the wall. Use as much weight as you can, without pushing back into the wall.

3. Roll down the wall until you are in a seated position, with knees at 90 degrees.

4. Roll back up. Do two or three sets of twenty reps each, or less if this is too much.

Lunge

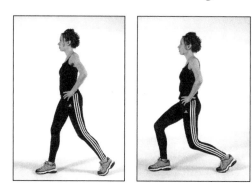

1. Stand straight, feet shoulder-width apart, with hands on hips.

2. Take a long step forward with your right foot. It should be flat on the floor. Your left foot should be on its ball.

3. Bend your left knee and lower your body, looking straight ahead with your body upright. Steps two and three are done in one motion.

4. Return to the starting position. Remember that your support leg knee should never extend past your toe. Repeat up to fifteen times on each leg.

Reverse Lunge

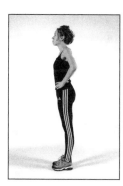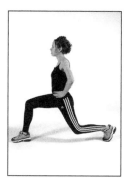

1. Stand straight, feet shoulder-width apart, with your hands on your hips.

2. Keeping your left leg straight, step back with your left foot as far as you can.

3. Lower your left knee as low as you can. Your right knee should be bent at a 90-degree angle. Steps two and three are done in one motion.

4. Lift yourself back to the starting position, tightening your bottom. Repeat ten times and then do the same with your right leg.

Side Leg Raises with Band

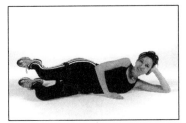 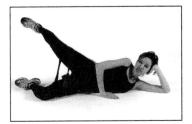

1. Tie the band around your thighs just above the knees. You will want the band tight enough to really feel the resistance.

2. Lie on one side with knees bent and heels lined up with your bottom. Be sure to keep your toes and knees facing forward.

3. Slowly raise and lower the upper leg, keeping knee in line with foot. Do two sets of fifteen reps. Repeat with other leg.

Knee Press with Band

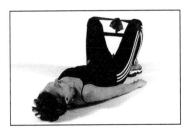

1. Sit down and tie band across your knees.

2. Lie down on your back on a mat or towel with your knees bent and your feet together, flat on the floor.

3. Press against the band by pushing outward with your knees.

4. Pause, then bring knees together. Remember to keep your pelvis up. Do up to three sets of fifteen reps, resting a few seconds between sets.

Hamstring Ball

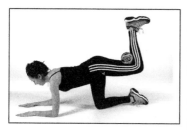

1. Get on elbows and knees, with ball or a five-pound weight behind your left knee, elbows under shoulders.

2. Lift your left leg to hip level, back straight, stomach tight, no twist in hips.

3. Pulse leg up and down, foot flexed, with ball in position. This is a small movement.

4. Switch legs and repeat. Do each leg up to twenty times.

The following thigh exercises can be done with or without a band or tubing. Or you can use ankle weights instead of a band or tubing. Do these every day without weights, or every other day with weights or bands.

Quad Lift

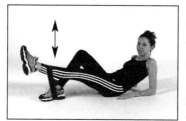

1. Tie the ends of the band together, giving yourself less tension at first—adjust tension as you progress.

2. Lie back, one foot flat on floor, the other extended in front of your body, resting on your elbows with lower back pressed to ground.

3. Loop the band around one ankle and hold it down with the other foot, as shown.

4. Slowly lift straight leg up as high as opposite knee.

5. Return to starting position and repeat, doing three sets of fifteen reps. Repeat with other leg.

Knee Extensions

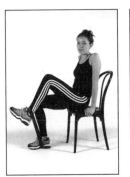

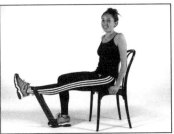

1. Tie ends of band together.

2. Sit up straight on a chair or bench, one foot flat on floor, the other leg bent and lifted toward chest.

3. Loop the band around one ankle and hold it down with the other foot.

4. Slowly straighten the knee without dropping the leg, but do not lock the knee.

5. Return to starting position and repeat, doing three sets of fifteen reps. Repeat with other leg.

Bottom Lift

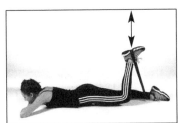

1. Lie on your stomach, one knee bent with ankle flexed, and heel toward your bottom.

2. Put the band on the foot of the pushing up leg and around the ankle on the anchor leg.

3. Tighten your bottom, lift the bent leg slightly off the ground and press your flexed foot toward the ceiling. Do not arch your back. Keep your hips on the ground.

4. Return to starting position and repeat, doing three sets of ten to fifteen reps, if you can. Repeat with the other leg.

Hamstring Curl

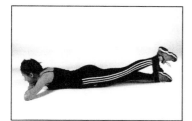 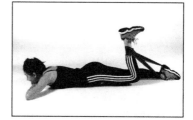

1. Lie on your stomach, tightening your bottom.

2. Bend one knee to lift your leg slightly off the ground. Put the band around your ankle on the curling leg and around your foot on the anchor leg.

3. While holding this position, slowly curl your heel toward your bottom. Keep your hips on the ground and do not arch your back.

4. Return to starting position and repeat, doing three sets of ten to fifteen reps. Repeat with other leg.

Thigh Lift

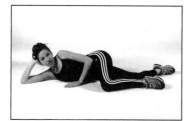 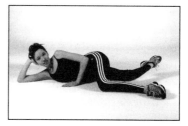

1. Lie on your side, with your head resting on your arm.

2. Your top leg should be bent and resting on the floor in front of your bottom leg, which is bent slightly. You can put a band around your thighs or ankles to increase intensity.

3. Lift your bottom leg, tightening your inner thigh. Continue lifting then lowering bottom leg without touching the ground. Be sure your hips and knees are forward. Repeat fifteen times, turn over and do the other leg.

Stretches

1. Make like a cat—get on your hands and knees and arch your back up.

2. Hold the stretch.

3. Sink your back down and hold the stretch. Repeat several times.

4. Sit on the floor with legs outstretched.

5. Pull one knee toward the chest and hug it, holding the stretch. Repeat with other leg.

6. Sit on the floor with your legs out straight.

7. Bend over slowly sliding your right hand past your right knee, towards your feet. Reach until you feel the stretch, don't bounce. Pause and repeat with left leg.

8. You may also do this exercise using a bench. Stand, put one leg straight out on the bench, lean forward and stretch, repeat on other leg.

It may take some practice to get these exercises down. But once you know how to do them and begin to do so on a regular basis, the rewards will soon become evident. If you work at the same time to increase your spiritual nourishment, as discussed in the next section of this book, you can achieve "mental and physical health and strength combined."

Brigham Young taught that "When you find the thinking faculty perfectly active, in a healthy person, it should put the physical organization into active operation, and the result of the reflection is carried out, and the object is accomplished. In such a person you will see mental and physical health and strength combined, in their perfection."[57]

SECTION THREE
Spiritual Nourishment

---14---

A SPIRITUAL DIET

*"Wherefore, verily I say unto you that all things
unto me are spiritual, and not at any time have I
given unto you a law which was temporal. . . . for
my commandments are spiritual."*

—*D&C 29:34–35*

The Word of Wisdom is not only a temporal, but also a
spiritual commandment. Following the Word of Wisdom
keeps your body healthy and creates a fitting environment
in which your spirit can dwell. The Word of Wisdom exem-
plifies the inextricable link between the body and the spirit,
as expressed in Doctrine and Covenants 88:15: "And the
spirit and the body are the soul of man" and in section 59,
verse 19, that God has provided "for food and for raiment,
for taste and for smell, to strengthen the body and to enliven
the soul." When I think of food with this dual purpose in
mind, it helps me make good choices about what I am going
to eat. I ask myself not just "What is this going to do for my
body?" but also, "What is this going to do for my spirit?"

Brigham Young explained: "So we see that almost the
very first teachings the first Elders of this Church received
were as to what to eat, what to drink, and how to order

their natural lives that they might be united temporally as well as spiritually. This is the great purpose which God has in view in sending to the world, by his servants, the Gospel of life and salvation."[58]

I am impressed by the depth of reasoning, spirituality, and purpose of the Word of Wisdom. The principles in the Word of Wisdom are truly part of the "Gospel of life and salvation."[59] Brigham Young put it this way: "Take care of yourselves, and live as long as you can, and do all the good you can."[60] On another occasion he further explained this important aspect of the Word of Wisdom: "Keep the Word of Wisdom—help the poor, feed the hungry, and clothe the naked."[61]

Brigham Young was concerned about the Saints' appetites and how they affected their ability to accomplish their purpose in life. He often had the dual meaning of *appetite* in mind when he cautioned the people: "The strength, power, beauty and glory that once adorned that form and constitution of man have vanished away before *the blighting influences of inordinate appetite and love of this world*. The health and power and beauty that once adorned the noble form of man must again be restored to our race."[62]

Brigham Young saw that the inability to control our appetite for food could be as deleterious to our spiritual health as to our physical health; that extravagant living would affect not just our spirits, but our bodies, rendering us spiritually numbed to and physically incapable of accomplishing our purposes in this life. "For as the body without the spirit is dead, so faith without works is dead also" (James 2:26).

The medical profession is more and more acknowledging the body-spirit connection to well-being. A newspaper article about a recent study published in *The Archives of Internal Medicine* states, "More than faith, it may be fact: Ill patients fare better when people pray for them, even when they're unaware that they're the subject of prayers, and even when they don't know the people doing the praying."[63]

Paul said, "I beseech you therefore, brethren, by the mercies of God, that ye present your bodies a living sacrifice, holy, acceptable unto God, which is your reasonable service" (Romans 12:1). In saying this, I think he meant that we should present healthy bodies, with healthy minds and spirits to God. Otherwise, how could our bodies be of service and a holy sacrifice to God?

Society spends a lot of time worrying about physical appearance. It is tied to self-esteem. But more important is our spiritual appearance. It *can* be seen, and it too is tied to our self-worth. Our spirits and bodies should be in a kind of "balance." Both need to be fed the right things. Brigham Young said: "You may take as much as you please of the Spirit of the Lord, and it will not make your stomach or head ache. You may drink nine cups of strong spiritual drink, and it will not hurt you; but if you drink nine cups of strong tea, see what it will do for you."[64]

To this point, this book has concentrated on building a strong body. As I close, we will focus on building a strong spirit. Your spirit needs nourishing, just as your body does. You probably already have in mind a weight goal. What is your spiritual goal? If you haven't yet, now is a good time to ask the Lord in prayer, "What am I to accomplish in my life and how can I best serve thee?" The scriptures give us plenty of ideas for constructing spiritual goals. Some of my favorites are in section 88 of the Doctrine and Covenants because I clearly see in them a temporal-spiritual link. These and other scriptures assist me with my spiritual diet. They are as follows:

• "And as all have not faith, seek ye diligently and teach one another words of wisdom; yea, seek ye out of the best books words of wisdom; seek learning, even by study and also by faith" (v. 118).

- "Organize yourselves; prepare every needful thing; and establish a house, even a house of prayer, a house of fasting, a house of faith, a house of learning, a house of glory, a house of order, a house of God" (v. 119).

- "Therefore, cease from all your light speeches, . . . from all your lustful desires, from all your pride and light-mindedness, and from all your wicked doings" (v. 121).

- "See that ye love one another; cease to be covetous; learn to impart one to another as the gospel requires" (v. 123).

- "Cease to be idle; cease to be unclean; cease to find fault one with another; cease to sleep longer than is needful; retire to thy bed early, that ye may not be weary; arise early, that your bodies and your minds may be invigorated" (v. 124).

- "And above all things, clothe yourselves with the bond of charity, as with a mantle, which is the bond of perfectness and peace" (v. 125).

- "Pray always" (v. 126).

Another of my favorite scriptures in the Doctrine and Covenants pertains to how we should approach our temporal and spiritual diet: "Let thy food be prepared with singleness of heart . . . that thy joy may be full. . . . And inasmuch as ye do these things with thanksgiving, with cheerful hearts and countenances, . . . the fulness of the earth is yours . . . for the benefit and the use of man, both to please the eye and to gladden the heart" (D&C 59:13–18).

When you sit down to eat, take a moment to give thanks for your food. Think about the blessings of good food and its purposes, and all the other blessings you have. Ponder the Word of Wisdom. Brigham Young said in reference to the Word of Wisdom, "There is life, everlasting life in it—the life which now is and the life which is to come."[65]

FURNISHING A SPIRITUAL HOME

*"As valuable as the Word of Wisdom is as a law
of health, it may be much more valuable to you
spiritually than it is physically."*

—*Boyd K. Packer*

Through the years I have lived all over the United States, in small rental apartments, little houses, and big houses. Each time I had the task of furnishing them as my financial circumstances permitted. I sometimes got very concerned about proper furniture placement, color scheme, and coordinating fabrics. I looked for a decorating theme for my home that would say, "This is Peggy." My physical surroundings often received more of my attention than did my spiritual surroundings. In truth, however, spiritual furnishings say more about us than any home decor can. Have you ever been in a home where the furniture did not match and the carpets were worn, but the home was warm and inviting and happy? By the same token, have you been in homes that were decorated to perfection, but felt cold and empty?

What is it that makes a home truly beautiful? Decorators often come into houses and perform what they call a "room-lift." They look at what is lacking, what does not go together, and what is placed incorrectly. Then they add, take away, and rearrange furnishings to try and create a harmonious effect. Pretend you are a decorator, but you want to give your home a "spiritual lift." What needs to be added, discarded, or rearranged so that your home is more harmonious and open to Heavenly Father's spirit? Every home needs these basic spiritual furnishings: prayer, faith, learning, honesty, order, service, and love. You can discard improper pride, extravagance, selfishness, destructive criticism, and discord. For your final touches, rearrange your priorities. In doing these things, you are likely to see the temporal things you are working on—maybe even your desire to lose weight—resolved as well.

Now let's look more closely at some of the basic spiritual furnishings.

PRAYER

"Evening, and morning, and at noon, will I pray, and cry aloud: and he shall hear my voice" (Psalm 55:17). "Counsel with the Lord in all thy doings, and he will direct thee for good; yea, when thou liest down at night lie down unto the Lord, that he may watch over you in your sleep; and when thou risest in the morning let thy heart be full of thanks unto God; and if ye do these things, ye shall be lifted up at the last day" (Alma 37:37).

I especially like the phrase "counsel with the Lord." It tells me that prayer is not a one-way mode of conversation. It also suggests that we can take our problems and concerns to Heavenly Father and reason with him. He will advise us and strengthen us.

Daily individual and family prayer can make all the difference in the atmosphere of our home. Surely, no home should be without it.

FAITH

Faith is not a theoretical construct. If it were, it would not make a difference in our lives. It does make a difference because it is real and it works. It makes the impossible possible, with God's help. "Yea, and how is it that ye have forgotten that the Lord is able to do all things according to his will, for the children of men, if it so be that they exercise faith in him?" (1 Nephi 7:12). In Hebrews, chapter 11, Paul explains, "Now faith is the substance of things hoped for, the evidence of things not seen" (v. 1). The entire chapter deals with faith, by which the world was made, miracles were wrought, and by which we can understand the works of God. A home without faith is a home without hope. In the trying times that come to every family, it is faith and hope that will see the family through and bring peace to the home.

LEARNING

"Give instruction to a wise man, and he will be yet wiser: teach a just man, and he will increase in learning. The fear of the Lord is the beginning of wisdom: and the knowledge of the holy is understanding" (Proverbs 9:9–10). We can make our homes places where learning of God and his commandments is an important part of the education of our children and ourselves. We can start by reading and discussing the scriptures together. Spiritual learning will bring an added dimension to secular learning. Our homes can also be places where we learn about nations, cultures, politics, people, science, art, music, and any other worthy pursuit. While television sometimes provides learning opportunities, the best thing you can do to increase learning in your home is to keep it off most of the time. Regardless of your age, you can increase your knowledge. Take time to further your own education. Keep current with world events and trends and read good literature.

Children are quick and eager learners. Even when children are quite small, they can be shown pictures in the newspaper and have the stories explained to them. Read to

them every day. In the past two years we have read as a
family *Treasure Island, The Adventures of Huckleberry Finn,
White Fang, Sounder, The Phantom Toll Booth,* and others. And
we have on hand ready to read *My Side of the Mountain, Call
of the Wild,* and *Tom Sawyer.* Classics like these really beat
watching television. Find out your children's interests and
talents and encourage them. I am lucky that I am a stay-at-
home mom. It makes it easier to provide learning opportunities for myself as well as for my son, simply because I
have more time. Shortly before the beginning of summer
vacation, I sit down with my son and we talk about the
things we want to learn that summer. We have science days,
art days, and so on. Make it obvious by your words and
choices that learning is important.

HONESTY

"Lying lips are abomination to the Lord: but they that
deal truly are his delight" (Proverbs 12:22). It is not easy for
children to learn honesty and integrity these days. Political
leaders, sports heroes, and other role models constantly dis-
appoint us and our children with their lack of honesty and
integrity. Cheating in schools and colleges is epidemic. The
Internet is making it easier than ever. It is not just the students who cheat. I remember not long ago reading about
the principal of a high school who had altered his school's
SAT scores to make it look as though his students were
doing better than they actually were.

I learned honesty from my parents. Your children should
learn it from you. Growing up we knew that dishonesty in
any form was abhorrent. We would sooner have contracted
leprosy than be caught cheating, it was that loathsome.
Never did I see my parents lie about our ages to get us
cheaper meals, movie tickets, or anything else. Never did I
see them keep the change when someone undercharged
them. It was not done and that was that.

ORDER

"Set in order your houses; keep slothfulness and uncleanness far from you" (D&C 90:18). A spiritually furnished home is neat and clean and in it respect for property is taught. Rules are agreed upon and enforced. A home where everyone is coming and going and no one seems to know what is going on or where anyone is is not an orderly home. I do not mean your home should be run like a military base, but if a home is chaotic, it is hard for the Spirit to dwell there. The Lord told Joseph Smith, "Behold, mine house is a house of order . . . and not a house of confusion" (D&C 132:8). I have heard some women talk of their disorganized home life as though the free-for-all contributed to a creative atmosphere for their children. Of course an *overly* regulated home can be stifling; but I have read enough parenting books and taken enough parenting classes to know that children thrive in a setting where they understand what is expected of them and what their boundaries are. Children need a sense of continuity and purpose. No wonder one of the definitions of "order" in Webster's New World Dictionary is "a state of peace and serenity." Isn't that the feeling we want in our home?

There are many other aspects of an orderly home, and an important one is financial order. Prophets through the ages have counseled us to get out of debt, and with good reason. Nothing is so grinding and destructive of peace and contentment in the home as excessive debt. In the Doctrine and Covenants, debt is described as "bondage" (19:35). In Proverbs we are told that if we are in debt we are servants "to the lender" (22:7). It is unfortunate that a common reason for debt is greed and a desire to appear prosperous and successful. But even if we are not living beyond our means, we can be too focused on material things. A friend who works with a financial institution gave me this sound advice for living providently and staying out of financial trouble: "Buy less. Stay out of malls. Buy one step down from what you think you can afford."

Finally, do not try to do too much. We can stress ourselves out by saying yes to too many things. Sometimes we act as though we can control the number of hours in a day. We suffer spiritually and emotionally and so does our family when we take on more than we can reasonably and successfully handle. "And see that all these things are done in wisdom and order; for it is not requisite that a man should run faster than he has strength" (Mosiah 4:27). In other words, do what you can and don't agonize over what you cannot do.

SERVICE

One of my favorite scriptures is Joshua 24:15. "Choose you this day whom ye will serve; . . . but as for me and my house, we will serve the Lord." Start early teaching your children the concept of service. They will learn by your example. Practice it first in your home by helping each other, and extend service from there. When we serve others we serve God: "Inasmuch as ye have done it unto one of the least of these my brethren, ye have done it unto me" (Matthew 25:40). Before Christmas I saw a neighbor and her children with two shopping carts full of food, clothes, and toys. "Boy, that's a big shop," I remarked. "We're doing Sub for Santa," one of the children answered. What a wonderful principle she was teaching her children!

Americans have been historically generous, but there are disturbing signs that this is changing. The gap between rich and poor in this country is widening. The 1999 Christmas season saw charitable donations go down. Experts attributed the drop in giving to the notion that the economy had been so good that people assumed everyone was prospering.

"But ye will teach them [children] to walk in the ways of truth and soberness; ye will teach them to love one another, and to serve one another. And also, ye yourselves will succor those that stand in need of your succor; ye will administer of your substance unto him that standeth in need" (Mosiah 4:15–16). There are many ways to serve others. Sometimes kind words and deeds are all that are necessary. When I was a single mother living in Virginia, and my older children were small, I was trying to think of ways to keep them occupied on Sundays while still keeping the Sabbath day holy. I had the idea of calling a nursing home in our neighborhood. Soon part of Sunday afternoon was spent visiting three of the most delightful women I have ever met. My children still vividly remember those sweet women.

I think fondly of a neighbor we had in Provo, Utah. Every heavy snowstorm he and his son would be out with the snow blower, clearing the sidewalks of the entire neighborhood. That family practiced service in more ways than I can count, and they were an example to everyone who knew them.

LOVE

Nothing furnishes a spiritual home so beautifully as love. "God is love; and he that dwelleth in love dwelleth in God, and God in him" (1 John 4:16). When there is love at home, everything else seems to fall into place. If you are married, one of the biggest favors you can do for your children is to let them see that you and your husband love each other. "Live joyfully with the wife whom thou lovest" (Ecclesiastes 9:9). Do you remember the story in Genesis of Jacob and Rachel? Her father required that Jacob work for him for seven years in order to marry Rachel. "And Jacob served seven years for Rachel; and they seemed unto him but a few days, for the love he had to her" (Genesis 29:20).

Love can work miracles in a home. The difficulty is that sometimes when your children (or spouse) seem to deserve it the least, they need it the most. It becomes easier if you think of it this way: love is given; it does not have to be earned. I was once told that I could do more to condition the standards around me than anyone else could. I have seen this truth played out many times. My mood and my attitude usually determine the tone of our home. I have to remind myself often that "love covereth all sins" (Proverbs 10:12) and that "a soft answer turneth away wrath" (Proverbs 15:1).

We also need to remember to love the *right* things. I was taught the following by a wise professor. It is a principle we should learn and teach to our children: "People are more important than things." With this concept as the bedrock of our thoughts and actions, we will see a big change in ourselves and in our families. Finally, as you contemplate what you can do to have a loving home, remember: "Better is a dinner of herbs where love is, than a stalled ox and hatred therewith" (Proverbs 15:17).

I am sure there are other spiritual furnishings that you would like to add to your home. You may want to pray about what should be added to your home, what should be discarded, and what should be rearranged. Talk about the spiritual "room-lift" for your home with family members and get their ideas. And take time to nourish your spirit. In doing so comes the solution to things both temporal and spiritual.

SECTION FOUR

Appendixes

A

NUTRITION WEB SITES AND ADDRESSES

WEB SITES

www.fns.usda.gov/fncs This site is sponsored by the Food, Nutrition, and Consumer Services division of the United States Department of Agriculture and provides diet and health information.

www.usda.gov/cnpp This site contains the Agriculture Center for Nutrition Policy and Promotion's "Healthy Eating and Dietary Guidelines" as well as links to the USDA's Food Guide Pyramid.

www.fda.gov This is the main page for United States Food and Drug Administration.

www.netwellness.com This site is maintained by the University of Cincinnati, Ohio State University, and Case Western Reserve University and is devoted to consumer health information.

www.healthfinder.gov The United States Department of Health and Human Services runs this site, providing links and searching mechanisms for health information and statistics.

www.eatright.org This is the Web site for the American Dietetic Association.

www.nih.gov/niams This site contains information about arthritis and osteoporosis, including their relationship to nutrition. It is run by the National Institute of Arthritis and Musculoskeletal and Skin Diseases.

www.nci.nih.gov This is the National Cancer Institute's Web site.

www.nhlbi.nih.gov This is the National Heart, Lung, and Blood Institute's Web site. It provides helpful information on cholesterol and obesity.

www.niddk.nih.gov/health/nutrit/win.htm This link will take you to the Weight Control Information Network and a plethora of valuable brochures, statistics, and credible weight loss information.

vm.cfsan.fda.gov/list.html This is the site for the Center for Food Safety and Applied Nutrition

www.niddk.nih.gov/health/nutrit/nutrit.htm This site contains publications, news releases and related links to health and nutrition information. It is run by the National Institute of Diabetes and Digestive and Kidney Diseases.

www.wfds.com The Worthington Foods Web site provides information and products for vegetarians or those wishing to find meat substitutes.

www.5aday.com This site, run by the Produce for Better Health Foundation and National Cancer Institute, provides information, programs, education, and recipes for children.

www.ext.usu.edu This is the Utah State University Extension Web site. It offers valuable nutrition information, including recipes.

ADDRESSES

United States Department of Agriculture
Center for Nutrition Policy and Promotion
1120 20th Street NW
Suite 200 North Lobby
Washington, DC 20036–3475

National High Blood Pressure Education Program
P.O. Box 30105
Bethesda, MD 20824–0105

"Healthy Eating for a Healthy Life"
AARP
Fulfillment, 601 E Street, NW
Washington, DC 20049

Weight Control Information Network
1 Win Way
Bethesda, MD 20892–3665

National Heart, Lung and Blood Institute Information Center
P.O. Box 30105
Bethesda, MD 20824–0105

B

VITAMINS AND MINERALS FOUND IN FRUITS

Fruit	Vitamin C	Vitamin A	Potassium
Apples	✓		
Apricots		✓	✓
Bananas	✓		✓
Blueberries	✓		
Cantaloupe	✓	✓	✓
Cherries			✓
Cranberries	✓		
Dates	✓		
Figs			✓
Grapefruit	✓		
Grapes	✓		
Guava fruit	✓	✓	✓
Honeydew melon	✓		✓
Kiwifruit	✓		✓
Mangoes	✓	✓	
Nectarines	✓	✓	✓
Oranges	✓		✓
Papayas	✓	✓	✓
Peaches	✓	✓	
Pears	✓		
Pineapple	✓		
Plums	✓		

Fruit	Vitamin C	Vitamin A	Potassium
Prickly pears	✓		
Prunes			✓
Raisins	✓		
Raspberries	✓		
Star fruit	✓	✓	
Strawberries	✓		
Tangerines	✓	✓	
Ugli fruit	✓		
Watermelon	✓	✓	

VITAMINS AND MINERALS FOUND IN VEGETABLES

Dark Green and Leafy Vegetables

Vegetable	Vitamin A	Vitamin C	Vitamin B₆	Calcium	Folate	Iron	Magnesium	Niacin	Potassium	Riboflavin	Zinc
Beet greens	✓	✓		✓	✓	✓	✓	✓	✓	✓	
Broccoli	✓	✓		✓	✓	✓	✓	✓	✓	✓	
Chard	✓	✓		✓	✓	✓	✓	✓	✓	✓	
Chicory	✓	✓		✓	✓	✓	✓	✓	✓	✓	
Collard greens	✓	✓		✓	✓	✓	✓	✓	✓	✓	
Dandelion greens	✓	✓		✓	✓	✓	✓	✓	✓	✓	
Endive	✓	✓		✓	✓	✓	✓	✓	✓	✓	
Escarole	✓	✓		✓	✓	✓	✓	✓	✓	✓	
Kale	✓	✓		✓	✓	✓	✓	✓	✓	✓	
Mustard green	✓	✓		✓	✓	✓	✓	✓	✓		
Romaine lettuce	✓	✓		✓	✓	✓	✓	✓	✓	✓	
Spinach	✓	✓		✓	✓	✓	✓	✓	✓	✓	
Turnip greens	✓	✓		✓	✓	✓	✓	✓	✓	✓	
Watercress	✓	✓		✓	✓	✓	✓	✓	✓	✓	

Deep Yellow Vegetables

Vegetable	Vitamin A	Vitamin C	Vitamin B₆	Calcium	Folate	Iron	Magnesium	Niacin	Potassium	Riboflavin	Zinc
Carrots	✓										
Pumpkin	✓										
Sweet Potatoes	✓										
Winter squash	✓										

Starchy Vegetables

Vegetable	Vitamin A	Vitamin C	Vitamin B₆	Calcium	Folate	Iron	Magnesium	Niacin	Potassium	Riboflavin	Zinc
Breadfruit			✓					✓	✓		✓
Corn			✓					✓	✓		✓
Green peas			✓					✓	✓		✓
Hominy			✓					✓	✓		✓
Lima beans			✓					✓	✓		✓
Potatoes			✓					✓	✓		✓
Rutabaga			✓					✓	✓		✓
Taro			✓					✓	✓		✓

Other Vegetables

Vegetable	Vitamin A	Vitamin C	Vitamin B6	Calcium	Folate	Iron	Magnesium	Niacin	Potassium	Riboflavin	Zinc
Artichokes	✓	✓							✓		
Asparagus	✓	✓							✓		
Bean and alfalfa sprouts	✓	✓							✓		
Beets	✓	✓							✓		
Brussels sprouts	✓	✓							✓		
Cabbage	✓	✓							✓		
Cauliflower											
Celery	✓	✓							✓		
Chinese cabbage	✓	✓							✓		
Cucumbers	✓	✓							✓		
Eggplant	✓	✓							✓		
Green beans	✓	✓							✓		
Green peppers	✓	✓							✓		
Lettuce	✓	✓							✓		

Vegetable	Vitamin A	Vitamin C	Vitamin B$_6$	Calcium	Folate	Iron	Magnesium	Niacin	Potassium	Riboflavin	Zinc
Mushrooms	✓	✓							✓		
Okra	✓	✓							✓		
Onions (mature and green)	✓	✓							✓		
Radishes	✓	✓							✓		
Snow peas	✓	✓							✓		
Summer squash	✓	✓							✓		
Tomatoes	✓	✓							✓		
Turnips	✓	✓							✓		
Vegetable juices	✓	✓							✓		
Zucchini	✓	✓							✓		

D

HINTS FOR REDUCING FAT, CHOLESTEROL, SUGAR, AND SODIUM IN YOUR BAKING

You can easily reduce the amount of fattening ingredients in your recipes or replace them with healthier substitutes. The following chart will give you some examples.

For	Use
1 whole egg	2 egg whites
whole milk	skim or lowfat milk
1 cup sugar	$\frac{1}{2}$ cup of sugar per cup of flour in cakes 1 tablespoon of sugar per cup of flour in yeast breads Hint: when reducing sugar, add more flavoring, such as vanilla
1 oz. baking chocolate	3 tablespoons of cocoa (if fat is needed, use 1 tablespoon or less of oil)
fat (any kind: butter, shortening, oil, etc.)	Use the minimual amount necessary and replace remainder with applesauce. minimum for muffins and quick breads is 1 to 2 tablespoons of fat per cup of flour minimum for cakes is 2 tablespoons of fat per cup of flour
sour cream	low-fat sour cream or yogurt

For	Use
sodium	¹/₄ teaspoon of salt per cup of flour in yeast breads; half the amount of salt called for in other baked products 1¹/₄ teaspoons of baking powder per cup of flour in muffins, biscuits, waffles 1 teaspoon of baking powder per cup of flour in cakes
butter	margarine or vegetable oil (total fat will be the same, but saturated fat and cholesterol will be reduced)

Source: *Food Facts for Older Adults,* United States Department of Agriculture, 1993, p. 40.

MODIFYING YOUR RECIPES

Here is an example of how to use the tips given in appendix D. The recipe below shows simple adjustments in a typical beef stroganoff recipe that can help you moderate fat and cholesterol.

Light Beef Stroganoff

$^3/_4$ pound beef round steak, boneless, trimmed*
$^1/_4$ pound fresh mushrooms
$^1/_2$ cup onion, sliced
$^1/_2$ cup beef broth, condensed
$^1/_2$ cup water

1 tablespoon catsup
$^1/_8$ teaspoon pepper
2 tablespoons flour
1 cup buttermilk*
2 cups noodles, cooked, unsalted (about $2^1/_2$ cups uncooked)

Slice steak across the grain into thin strips, about $^1/_8$-inch wide and 3 inches long. (It is easier to cut thin slices of meat if it is partially frozen.)

Wash and slice mushrooms.

Cook beef strips, mushrooms, and onion in nonstick* frypan until beef is lightly browned.

Add broth, water, catsup, and pepper. Cover and simmer until beef is tender, about 45 minutes.

Mix flour with about $^1/_4$ cup of the buttermilk* until smooth; add remaining buttermilk. Stir into beef mixture. Cook, stirring constantly, until thickened.

Serve over noodles. Makes 4 half-cup servings.

Each serving provides: 275 calories, 6 g total fat, 2 g saturated fatty acids, 71 mg cholesterol, 325 mg sodium.

*CHANGES FROM TYPICAL RECIPE

1. Use a less fatty meat cut—round steak in place of sirloin—and trim fat from meat.

2. Use buttermilk in place of sour cream.

3. Use a non-stick pan and no butter to cook the meat.

4. Prepare gravy with buttermilk instead of butter.

For each serving, these changes result in savings of 240 calories, 24 grams total fat, 15 grams saturated fatty acids, and 62 milligrams cholesterol.

Source: *Food Facts for Older Adults,* United States Department of Agriculture, 1993, p. 65.

ADAPTING YOUR STAPLES

You can reduce fat and sodium in the boxed products you use, such as macaroni and cheese. Just follow the chart below:

Mix	Changes	Fat saved (per serving)	Sodium saved (per serving)
Macaroni and cheese (³/₄ cup serving)	• Omit salt when cooking. • Use lowfat milk. • Reduce added margarine by half.	6 g	265 mg
Seasoned rice and rice/pasta mixes (¹/₂ cup serving)	• Reduce added margarine by half.	2 g	20 mg
Bread stuffing (¹/₂ cup serving)	• Reduce added margarine by half.	4 g	45 mg
Scalloped and au gratin potatoes (¹/₂ cup serving)	• Use lowfat milk. • Reduce addedmargarine by half.	2 g	20 mg

Note: Savings for macaroni and cheese and potatoes are for products made with 2 percent fat milk in place of whole milk. Reduce fat even further by using 1 percent fat or skim milk.

Source: *Food Facts for Older Adults*, United States Department of Agriculture, 1993, p. 66.

─── G ───
HOW DO YOU SCORE ON SODIUM?

	Seldom or never	1 to 2 times a week	3 to 5 times a week	Almost daily
How often do you—				
1. Eat cured or processed meats, such as ham, sausage, frankfurters, and other luncheon meats?	❑	❑	❑	❑
2. Choose canned vegetables or frozen vegetables with sauce?	❑	❑	❑	❑
3. Use frozen TV dinners, entrees, or canned or dehydrated soups?	❑	❑	❑	❑
4. Eat cheese?	❑	❑	❑	❑
5. Eat salted nuts, popcorn, pretzels, corn chips, or potato chips?	❑	❑	❑	❑
6. Add salt to cooking water for vegetables, rice, pasta, or cereals, or add seasoning mixes or sauces containing salt when preparing foods?	❑	❑	❑	❑
7. Salt your food before tasting it?	❑	❑	❑	❑

Several checks in the last two columns mean you may have a high sodium intake. Perhaps you could use those types of foods less often, or in smaller quantities. Watching your sodium can be a real challenge at certain meals or snacks.

Source: *Food Facts for Older Adults,* United States Department of Agriculture, 1993, p. 12

—————— H ——————

HOW DO YOU SCORE ON FAT?

	Seldom or never	1 to 2 times a week	3 to 5 times a week	Almost daily
How often do you eat—				
1. Fried, deep-fat fried, or breaded foods?	❑	❑	❑	❑
2. Fatty meats, such as sausage, luncheon meats, fatty steaks and roasts?	❑	❑	❑	❑
3. Whole milk, high-fat cheeses, ice cream?	❑	❑	❑	❑
4. Pies, pastries, rich cakes?	❑	❑	❑	❑
5. Rich cream sauces and gravies?	❑	❑	❑	❑
6. Oily salad dressings, mayonnaise?	❑	❑	❑	❑
7. Butter or margarine on vegetables, dinner rolls, toast?	❑	❑	❑	❑

Several checks in the last two columns mean you may have a high fat intake. Perhaps you could use those types of foods less often, or in smaller quantities. Watching your fat can be a real challenge at certain meals or snacks.

Source: *Food Facts for Older Adults,* United States Department of Agriculture, 1993, p. 11.

I

ARE YOU GETTING ENOUGH FIBER IN YOUR DIET?

	Seldom or never	1 to 2 times a week	3 to 5 times a week	Almost daily
How often do you eat—				
1. Three or more servings of breads and cereals made with whole grains?	❑	❑	❑	❑
2. Starchy vegetables such as potatoes, corn, peas, or dishes made with dry beans or peas?	❑	❑	❑	❑
3. Several servings of other vegetables?	❑	❑	❑	❑
4. Whole fruit with skins and/or seeds (berries, apples, pears, etc.)?	❑	❑	❑	❑

The best answer is Almost Daily. Whole-grain products, fuits, and vegetables provide fiber. Eating a variety of these foods daily will provide you with adequate fiber, both soluble and insoluble types.

Source: *Food Facts for Older Adults,* United States Department of Agriculture, 1993, p. 23.

J

FIBER IN FOODS

Food	Serving size	Grams of dietary fiber (soluble & insoluble)
Fruits		
Apple, with skin	1 medium	2.0-2.5
Banana	1 medium	1.8
Blueberries	½ cup	1.7
Cantaloupe	¼	1.1
Figs, dried	2	3.5
Grapes, seedless	½ cup	1.0
Grapefruit, white or pink	½	1.6
Kiwi	1	2.6
Orange	1 medium	3.1
Peach, with skin	1 medium	1.4
Pear, with skin	1 medium	4.3
Pineapple, fresh or canned	½ cup	1.2
Prunes, dried	3	1.8
Raisins, seedless	¼ cup	1.9
Strawberries	1 cup	3.9
Watermelon	1 cup	0.6

Vegetables, cooked

Asparagus, cooked from frozen	½ cup	1.6
Broccoli, cooked from frozen	½ cup	2.5
Brussels sprouts, cooked from fresh or frozen	½ cup	3.4
Corn, cooked from frozen	½ cup	3.4
Green beans, cooked from frozen	½ cup	2.1
Onion, cooked from fresh	½ cup	1.5
Potato, baked, with skin	1 medium	3.6
Spinach, cooked from frozen	½ cup	2.5

Food	Serving size	Grams of dietary fiber (soluble & insoluble)
Sweet potato, baked in skin	1 medium	3.4
Zucchini, cooked from fresh	½ cup	1.8

Vegetables, raw

Cabbage, shredded	1 cup	1.7
Carrots	1 medium	2.3
Cauliflower	½ cup	1.3
Celery	1 stalk	0.6
Cucumber, sliced	½ cup	0.5
Lettuce, romaine	1 cup	1.0
Mushrooms, sliced	½ cup	1.5
Spinach as salad greens	1 cup	1.9
Tomato	1 medium	1.6

Legumes, cooked

Baked beans, canned	½ cup	7.0
Black beans	½ cup	7.7
Black-eyed peas, canned	½ cup	8.5
Green peas, cooked from frozen	½ cup	3.6
Kidney beans	½ cup	7.3
Lentils	½ cup	3.7
Refried beans	½ cup	6.0
Soybeans, cooked from dry	½ cup	3.0

Breads, Grains, Pasta

Bagel	1	1.2
Bran muffin	1 medium size	2.8
Corn bread muffin	1 medium size	1.6
French bread	1 slice	0.8
Pumpernickel bread	1 slice	1.9
Rice, brown, cooked	½ cup	1.7
Rice, white, cooked	½ cup	0.0
Spaghetti	½ cup	1.6
Taco shell	1	1.1

Food	Serving size	Grams of dietary fiber (soluble & insoluble)
White bread	1 slice	0.5
Whole-wheat bread (100% whole-wheat)	1 slice	1.9

Snack Foods

Corn chips	1 ounce	1.3
Fig bar cookies	2 cookies	1.3
Graham crackers	2 crackers	0.6
Peanuts, dry roasted	$\frac{1}{4}$ cup	2.9
Popcorn, air-popped	1 cup	0.9
Rye crackers, whole grain	2 crackers	2.2
Sunflower seeds	$\frac{1}{4}$ cup	2.3
Walnuts, English	$\frac{1}{4}$ cup	1.4

Breakfast Cereals

See the Nutrition Facts label for the fiber content of your favorite cereal. If the label shows 10% of the Daily Value for fiber, this means that one serving contains 10% of the recommended 25 grams of fiber daily. To calculate grams of fiber in one serving: 10% x 25 grams = 2.5 grams of fiber.

Source: Washington State Dairy Council, 1996.

THE VEGETARIAN FOOD PYRAMID

A Daily Guide to Food Choices

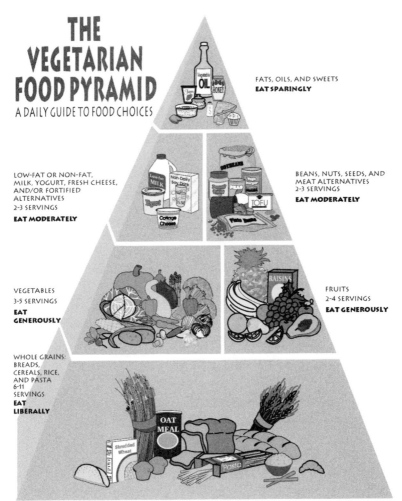

THE
**VEGETARIAN
FOOD PYRAMID**
A DAILY GUIDE TO FOOD CHOICES

FATS, OILS, AND SWEETS
EAT SPARINGLY

LOW-FAT OR NON-FAT,
MILK, YOGURT, FRESH CHEESE,
AND/OR FORTIFIED
ALTERNATIVES
2-3 SERVINGS
EAT MODERATELY

BEANS, NUTS, SEEDS, AND
MEAT ALTERNATIVES
2-3 SERVINGS
EAT MODERATELY

VEGETABLES
3-5 SERVINGS
**EAT
GENEROUSLY**

FRUITS
2-4 SERVINGS
EAT GENEROUSLY

WHOLE GRAINS:
BREADS,
CEREALS, RICE,
AND PASTA
6-11
SERVINGS
**EAT
LIBERALLY**

SOURCE: the Health Connection, (800) 548-8700, 1994.   ILLUSTRATION BY MERLE POIRIER

SPICE COMPATIBILITY CHART

Name	Description	Compatible with
Allspice (spice)	Whole or Ground *Color:* dried brown, pea-sized berries *Flavor:* spicy-sweet, mild, pleasant	Fruit compote, preserves, baked bananas, all cranberry dishes; spice cake, molasses cookies; beets, spinach, squash, turnips, red cabbage, carrots; green pea soup*; meat loaf, hamburgers, beef stew, baked ham, lamb, meat gravies*; mincemeat; boiled fish*; pickles*, pickle relishes; tapioca pudding, chocolate pudding.
Anise (seed)	Whole and Ground *Color:* brown with tan stripes *Flavor:* sweet licorice aroma and taste	Coffee cake*, sweet breads, rolls*, cookies*; fruit compote*, stewed apples*, preserved fruits*, all fruit pie fillings*; licorice candies; sweet pickles*; beef and veal stew*; cottage cheese.
Basil (herb)	Fresh or dried leaves and stems. *Color:* light green *Flavor:* pleasant, mild, sweet, distinctive	All tomato dishes, peas, squash, string beans, potatoes, spinach, French and Russian dressing or sprinkle over salads; bean soup, pea soup, beef soup, Manhattan clam chowder; broiled lamb chops, venison, beef, lamb and veal stews, veal roasts; shrimp, shrimp creole, boiled and steamed lobster, spaghetti sauce; scrambled eggs; souffles.

*The whole spice can be used.

Name	Description	Compatible with
Bay Leaves (herb)	Available as dried whole leaves. *Color:* light green *Flavor:* very mild, sweet, distinctive •Remove from dish and discard before serving	Pickled beets, beets, boiled carrots, boiled artichokes, boiled potatoes, vegetable soup, fish chowders; lamb, beef, veal, venison, poultry, fish stews; boiled or steamed shrimp and lobster; chicken casserole, boiled chicken; pickled meats; brine for smoked meats; pot roast; boiled pork; meat gravies; marinades.
Caraway (seed)	*Color:* dark brown with light brown stripes *Flavor:* tastes like rye bread; in fact, caraway gives rye bread its flavor	Mild cheese spreads, cream cheese, cottage cheese; bread, rolls, buns, muffins, coffee cake, cookies; cooked cabbage, cauliflower, potatoes, tomatoes, carrots, celery, onions, turnips, beets, broccoli, Brussels sprouts; cooked sauerkraut, cole slaw, salads, soup, sauerbraten, beef a la mode, roast pork, roast goose.
Cardamon (seed)	Whole and Ground *Color:* pod is cream colored, seeds dark brown *Flavor:* bitter-sweet, distinctive	Danish pastry, buns, coffee cake; grape jelly; custards; baked apple* fruit cup, sprinkled on chilled melon; sweet potato dishes, pumpkin pie, cookies, frozen ice cream, puddings.
Cayenne (spice)	Ground *Color:* burnt orange *Flavor:* hot	Deviled eggs; clam and oyster stews, poached salmon; seafood sauces, barbecue sauce for meat and fish; tuna fish salad; cottage and cream cheeses; cooked green vegetables; Welsh rarebit, cheese souffles; pork chops, veal stew, ham croquettes.

*The whole spice can be used.

Name	Description	Compatible with
Celery Seed (seed)	Whole *Color:* deep to light shades of brownish-green *Flavor:* bitter celery	Cream of celery soup, meat loaf, meat stews; fish chowders and stews; celery sauce, cole slaw, pickles; cabbage, turnips, braised lettuce, white potatoes, stewed tomatoes; rolls, biscuits, salty bread stuffings; eggs; salads and salad dressings.
Chili Powder (blend)	*Color:* ranges from light to dark red *Flavor:* distinctive	Mexican cookery, arroz con pollo, chili con carne; meat loaf, hamburgers, beef, pork, veal stew; shellfish, creamed seafood; boiled and scrambled eggs; cocktail sauces; Spanish rice, gravies, pepperpot soup; vegetable relishes, French dressing.
Cinnamon (spice)	Whole and Ground *Color:* light brown *Flavor:* distinctive, sweet, spicy	Buns, coffee cake, muffins, spice cake, molasses cookies, butter cookies, cinnamon toast, custards, tapioca, chocolate pudding, rice pudding, fruit pies, broiled grapefruit, apples in any form, stewed fruits*, pickled fruits*, heated spiced beverages, hot cocoa and chocolate drinks; sweet gherkins; sweet potatoes, pumpkin, squash.
Cloves (spice)	Whole and ground Color: dark brown Flavor: distinctive, spicy, sweet, penetrating	Ham*, pork roast*, pickled fruits*, preserved fruits*, stewed fruits*; apple, minced and pumpkin pies; beets, baked beans, candied sweet potatoes, squash; spice cake; sweet gherkin; rice pudding, chocolate pudding; tapioca; bean soup, beef soup, cream of pea soup, cream of tomato soup.
Red Pepper (spice)	*Color:* bright red to orange *Flavor:* hot	Pizzas, sausages, Italian specialties; whenever heat and spot color are desired.

*The whole spice can be used.

Name	Description	Compatible with
Cumin (seed)	Ground *Color:* gold with a hint of green *Flavor:* distinctive, salty-sweet, a principal flavoring ingredient of chili powder	Deviled eggs; cream, cottage and Cheddar cheeses*; meat loaf, hamburgers, chili con carne; fruit pies; cabbage*, rice; sauerkraut; fish.
Curry Powder (blend)	Color: varies depending on ingredients, predominately rich gold Flavor: distinctive, exotic, with heat depending on blend	Eggs, deviled eggs; fish; shrimp; poultry, chicken hash; meat; vegetables, rice, scalloped tomatoes, creamed vegetables, cottage and cream cheeses; French dressing, mayonnaise, white sauce; clam and fish chowders, tomato soup, cream of mushroom soup; salted nuts; sweet pickles.
Dill (seed)	Whole and Ground *Color:* dark purplish brown with tan stripes *Flavor:* similar to caraway, but milder and sweeter	Pickling*; sauerkraut; potato salad; macaroni, cottage and cream cheese; split pea soup, navy bean soup, cream of tomato soup, apple pie; broiled lamb chops, lamb stew, creamed chicken, French dressing; sour cream salad dressing; drawn butter for shellfish; spiced vinegar, peas, carrots, beets, cabbage, cauliflower, snap beans, turnips.
Fennel (seed)	Whole *Color:* light sand-colored seed with brown stripes *Flavor:* sweet licorice, mild, anise-like	Sweet pickles; boiled fish; bread, buns, coffee cake, muffins, sugar cookies, apples in any form; beef stew, squashes, roast pork.
Garlic (bulb)	Bulb *Color:* white *Flavor:* pungent	Any food where a garlic flavor is desired.
Garlic Powder (vegetable seasoning)	*Color:* white *Flavor:* garlic (product is result of dehydrating and grinding garlic). Contains no salt. Granulated garlic is similar product but more coarsely ground.	Wherever garlic is used.

*The whole spice can be used.

197

Name	Description	Compatible with
Ginger (spice)	Whole *Color:* tan *Flavor:* distinctive spicy, penetrating Ground *Color:* light tan *Flavor:* same as above	Cookies, spice cake, pumpkin pie; Indian pudding; baked, stewed and preserved fruits, apple sauce; custard; conserves, chutney; buttered beets, carrots, squash; poultry, broiled and chopped beef, lamb and veal, bean soup; pickles; baked beans; cheese dishes; meat stews; French dressing.
Horseradish (root)	Root *Color:* light brown *Flavor:* bitter, pungent	One of the five bitter herbs of passover. Use sparingly. Grate peeled, fresh root into lemon or vinegar. If using dried root, reconstitute not more than 30 minutes before serving. To reconstitute, grind and soak 1 tablespoon dried horseradish in 2 tablespoons water and add $^1/_2$ cup cream.
Mace (spice)	Whole or Ground *Color:* burnt orange *Flavor:* sweet, exotic aroma and strong nutmeg flavor	Fish sauces*, oyster and clam stews; creamed soups, pickling*, preserved fruits*; gingerbread batter; stewed cherries*, fruit salad*, sweet spiced doughs, doughnuts, light fruit cakes, pound cake; Welsh rarebit*; meat loaf, veal chops; all chocolate dishes; whipped cream; cottage pudding; custard, carrots, cauliflower, potatoes, spinach, succotash, fruit pies.
Marjoram (herb)	Whole and Ground *Color:* green *Flavor:* distinctive, delicate Fresh or dried	Lamb chops, roast beef, pork, veal, chicken, duck, goose; salmon loaf and other baked and broiled fish; omelets and souffles; tossed green salad; onion, clam, and oyster soups, stews; eggplant, carrots, peas, spinach, stuffings.

*The whole spice can be used.

Name	Description	Compatible with
Mint, peppermint, spearmint (herb)	Whole or Flaked *Color:* green *Flavor:* distinctive, sweet aroma	Jelly, ice cream, custard, fruit salad, fruit compote; frostings; split pea soup; lamb and veal roast sauces; cottage cheese salad; white potatoes, cabbage, carrots, celery, snap beans; tea; mint sauce.
Mixed Pickling (blend of whole spices)	*Flavor:* in cooking, blend is distinctive, pleasant, spicy, and sweet	Pickles, relishes; preserves; gravies, meat stews, pork, veal, lamb, beef; cooked vegetables, boiled salmon; marinades; shrimp.
Mustard (spice)	Ground or Powdered *Color:* copper *Flavor:* distinctive, spicy, sharp (prepared mustard contains vinegar and oil mixed with mustard)	Pickles*, pickled onions*; salads*, salad dressings; pickled meats*; boiled fish*; Chinese hot sauce, fish sauces, cheese sauces; ham, kidneys; deviled eggs; creamed and stewed oysters, shrimp; asparagus, beets, broccoli, Brussels sprouts, cabbage, celery, onions, white potatoes, snap beans, squash; molasses cookies.
Nutmeg (spice)	Ground *Color:* copper *Flavor:* distinctive, exotic, sweet	Doughnuts; eggnog, custards, puddings, whipped cream, ice cream; fried bananas, stewed fruits; spice cake, coffee cake, cookies, pumpkin pie, steamed and glazed carrots, cabbage, spinach, snap beans, squash, onions, sweet potatoes; meat loaf.
Onion Powder (vegetable seasoning)	*Color:* white *Flavor:* onion (product is result of dehydrating and grinding onion.) Contains no salt. Granulated onion is similar product but more coarsely ground.	Wherever onion flavor is desired.
Onion Salt (vegetable seasoning)	*Color:* cream *Flavor:* similar to onion powder but much milder because of addition of salt	Wherever slight onion flavor is desired.

*The whole spice can be used.

Name	Description	Compatible with
Onion, minced (vegetable seasoning)	Dehydrated minced *Color:* white *Flavor:* onion flavor	Wherever minced or finely chopped onion is used. Chives, allium, scallions are of this family.
Oregano (herb)	Whole and Ground *Color:* green *Flavor:* distinctive, strong Fresh or dried	Pizza, spaghetti sauce, meat sauce; Swiss steak, beef stew, broiled and roast lamb, pork and veal, poultry; gravies; stuffed fish; cheese spreads; beef soup, bean soup, tomato soup; butter sauce for shell-fish; cream and tomato sauces; vegetable juice cocktail, onions, peas, white potatoes, spinach, string beans.
Paprika (spice)	Ground *Color:* red *Flavor:* distinctive, very mild	Poultry, ham, goulash, fish, shellfish; salad dressings; veg-etables; gravies; cheese, Welsh rarebit; canapes; deviled eggs; stuffed celery, cream soups, chicken soup, chowders.
Parsley Flakes (herb)	*Color:* green *Flavor:* distinctive, mild Fresh or dried High in Vitamin A	Soups; salads; cole slaw; meat stews, fish, poultry; sauces; all vegetables; omelets; potatoes.
Black Pepper (spice)	Whole or Ground *Color:* dark brown *Flavor:* distinctive, pleas-ant spicy bouquet with palate-tingling flavor and enduring after-taste.	Almost all foods, except those with sweet flavors. If you are preparing a non-sweet dish that "needs something" try a little pepper first. It is used universally to add sparkle to foods, including: Pickles*; soups; poultry, meats*, fish*, shellfish, game, sauces, gravies, marinades; salads; eggs; cheese spreads, vegeta-bles; spiced vinegar.
White Pepper (spice)	Whole or Ground *Color:* varies from beige to brown *Flavor:* penetrating, strong with enduring after-taste	Same as above. White pepper is used where black specks are not desired, such as in white sauces, clear soups, mashed potatoes, etc.

*The whole spice can be used.

Name	Description	Compatible with
Poppy (seed)	Whole *Color:* predominantly blue gray *Flavor:* crunchy texture, nut-like	Breads, rolls, coffee cake, cookies, pie crusts; noodles; cottage cheese, salad dressing; green peas, white potatoes, rutabagas.
Rosemary (herb)	Whole *Color:* green (looks like a pine needle) *Flavor:* distinctive, delicate, sweetish	Roast and broiled lamb, beef, pork, veal, game, poultry; salmon; deviled eggs; cheese sauces; sauteed mushrooms, boiled potatoes, green peas, squash; creamed seafood; chicken soup; split pea soup.
Sage (herb)	Whole *Color:* olive green *Flavor:* distinctive, positive	All pork dishes; meat, fish and poultry stuffings; brown sauces; cheese spreads; consomme, cream soups, fish chowders; salad greens, French dressing; Brussels sprouts, onions, lima beans, peas, tomatoes.
Saffron (spice)	Whole and Ground *Color:* predominantly maroon *Flavor:* distinctive, exotic, concentrated (not strong, yet a little goes a long way)	Rice; rolls, breads, buns; fish stew; bouillabaisse chicken; chicken soup; cakes.
Savory (herb)	Whole and Ground *Color:* green *Flavor:* distinctive, pleasant, mild Winter and summer are different flavors.	Scrambled eggs, omelets, deviled eggs, liver pate, chicken loaf, poultry stuffing; hamburgers, lamb pie, veal roast, fish; tossed salad; lentil soup, consomme, fish chowder; beets, beans, cabbage, peas.
Sesame (seed)	*Color:* predominantly cream *Flavor:* crunchy texture sweet, decidedly nut-like	Rolls, breads, buns, cookies, coffee cakes, pies; soft cheeses; salad dressings, fish, asparagus, snap beans, tomatoes, candies. Increased flavor when toasted.

*The whole spice can be used.

Name	Description	Compatible with
Tarragon (herb)	Whole and Ground *Color:* green *Flavor:* distinctive, pleasant, fresh	Marinades for meat, butter sauce for steaks, poultry; salads; omelets, fish and shellfish; vegetable juice cocktail, chicken soup, consomme, fish chowder, tomato soup; vinegar; broccoli, asparagus, beans, cabbage, cauliflower.
Thyme (herb)	Whole and Ground *Color:* gray-green *Flavor:* distinctive, pleasantly penetrating A variety of flavor.	Fresh tomatoes, tomato aspic, salads; poultry stuffing, croquettes, fricassees; fish chowders, gumbo, vegetable soup, shirred eggs, all meats, seafood sauces; artichokes, beans, beets, carrots, mushrooms, onions, potatoes.
Turmeric (spice)	Whole and Ground *Color:* orange (used mostly for its color) *Flavor:* mild, slightly bitter	Pickles, relishes, prepared mustards, salad dressings; creamed eggs, fish, seafood; to color rice dishes where saffron is not used.

NOTES

Introduction

1. Daniel H. Ludlow, *A Companion to Your Study of the Doctrine and Covenants,* vol. 1 (Salt Lake City: Deseret Book Company, 1978), p. 463.
2. James E. Enstrom, "Health Practices and Cancer Mortality among Active California Mormons," in *Latter-day Saint Social Life,* ed. James T. Duke (Provo: Brigham Young University Religious Studies Center, 1998), pp. 441–60.
3. Bert Connell, personal interview with author, October 12, 1999. Dr. Bert Connell, Ph.D., R.D., is the chair of the Department of Nutrition and Dietetics at Loma Linda University.
4. Brigham Young, *Journal of Discourses,* 26 vols. (London: Latter-day Saints' Book Depot, 1854–86), 7:138.

Chapter 1

5. Brigham Young, *Journal of Discourses,* 12:156.
6. Brigham Young, *Journal of Discourses,* 13:153–54.
7. Brigham Young, *Journal of Discourses,* 4:103 and 6:148.

Chapter 2

8. Brigham Young, *Journal of Discourses,* 11:132.
9. "Top-selling Diets," *Consumer Reports,* January 1998, pp. 60–61.
10. Brigham Young, *Journal of Discourses,* 12:209.
11. Eugenia E. Calle, Michael J. Thun, Jennifer M. Petrelli, Carmen Rodriguez, and Clark W. Heath, Jr., " Body-Mass Index and Mortality in a Prospective Cohort of U.S. Adults," *New England Journal of Medicine* 341, no. 15 (1999): 1097–1105.
12. Ali H. Mokdad, Mary K. Serdula, William H. Dietz, Barbara

A. Bowman, James S. Marks, and Jeffrey P. Koplan, "The
Spread of the Obesity Epidemic in the United States,
1991–1998," *JAMA* 282, no. 16 (1999): 1519–22

13. *The Facts about Weight Loss Products and Programs* [brochure],
    Washington D.C.: U. S. Food and Drug Administration,
    1992; see also www.cfsan.fda.gov/~dms/wgtloss.html

14. Ibid.

15. Ibid.

16. Brigham Young, *Journal of Discourses*, 8:139, 141.

17. Brigham Young, *Journal of Discourses*, 12:122.

18. *Nutrition and Your Health: Dietary Guidelines for Americans* 4th
    ed. [brochure], Washington D.C.: United States Department
    of Agriculture, 1995; see also
    www.ars.usda.gov/dgac/dgacguidexp.htm

19. *Food Guide Pyramid* [brochure], United States Department of
    Agriculture, United States Department of Health and
    Human Services, 1992.

20. *Making Healthy Food Choices* [brochure], United States
    Department of Agriculture, Human Information Systems,
    1993.

Chapter 3

21. *Pyramid Plus: A Star-Studded Guide to Food Choices for Better
    Health* [brochure], Nutrition Education Services/Oregon
    Dairy Council, 1997. For more information about Pyramid
    Plus, call (503) 229-5033.

Chapter 4

22. Brigham Young, *Journal of Discourses*, 8:281.

23. *Do You Know the Health Risks of Being Overweight?* [brochure],
    Bethesda, Md.: National Institutes of Health, 1998; see also
    http://137.187.36.5/health/nutrit/pubs/health.htm#what
    or write to 1 Win Way Bethesda, MD 20892-3665.

24. JoAnn Manson, as quoted in Katharine Webster, "Excess Weight Kills, Obesity Study Finds," *Deseret News,* October 7, 1999, p. A8.

25. Ibid.

26. Brigham Young, *Journal of Discourses,* 12:122.

27. Brigham Young, *Journal of Discourses,* 19:68.

28. *Eating for Life* [brochure], Bethesda, Md.: National Institutes of Health, 1988.

29. Ibid.

30. Joshipura J. Kaumudi, Alberto Ascherio, JoAnn E. Manson, Meir J. Stampfer, Eric B. Rimm, Frank E. Speizer, Charles H. Hennekens, Donna Spiegelman, and Walter C. Willett, "Fruit and Vegetable Intake in Relation to Risk of Ischemic Stroke," *JAMA* 282, no. 13 (1999): 1233–39.

31. Jeffrey P. Koplan and William H. Dietz, "Caloric Imbalance and Public Health Policy," *JAMA* 282, no. 16 (1999): 1580.

32. Brigham Young, *Journal of Discourses,* 14:89; 2:269; 13:142; 12:37.

Chapter 5

33. *Weight Loss for Life* [brochure], Bethesda, Md.: National Institutes of Health, 1998; see also www.niddk.nih.gov/health/nutrit/pubs/wtloss/wtloss.htm or write to 1 Win Way Bethesda, MD 20892-3665.

Chapter 6

34. Richard P. Troiano and Katherine M. Flegal, "Overweight Children and Adolescents: Description, Epidemiology, and Demographics," *Pediatrics* 101, no. 3 (Supplment March 1998): 497–504.

35. Ruth Papazian, "On the Teen Scene: Should You Go on a Diet?" *FDA Consumer* 27 (September 1993): 31–33.

36. Catherine A. Tomeo, "Weight Concerns, Weight Control

Behaviors, and Smoking Initiation," *Pediatrics* 104 (October 1999): 918–925.

37. Stacey Schultz, "Why We're Fat: Gender and Age Matter More Than You May Realize," *U.S. News & World Report*, November 8, 1999, p. 83.

38. Ibid.

39. Ibid.

40. Sheila Ashbrook, *Sports Nutrition Member's Guide* (Urbana, Ill.: University of Illinois Cooperative Extension Service), 1997.

41. Stacey Schultz, "Why We're Fat," pp. 83–85.

42. Roberta Larson Duyff, *The American Dietetic Association's Complete Food & Nutrition Guide* (Minneapolis: Chronimed Publishing, 1996), p. 473.

43. Sarah Goodlin, personal interview with author, November 11, 1999.

Chapter 7

44. Joshipura J. Kaumudi, et al., "Fruit and Vegetable Intake," *JAMA* 282 (1999):1233–39.

45. Rebecca Low and Deloy Hendricks, *Food Storage Cooking School: "Use It or Lose It,"* 2d ed. (Salt Lake County: Utah State University Extension, 1999), pp. 8-20; see also www.ext.usu.edu/publica/foodpubs.htm

Chapter 8

46. Roberta Larson Duyff, *American Dietetic Association's Complete Food & Nutrition Guide*, p. 103.

47. Ralph E. Whitesides, *Home Storage of Wheat* (Logan, Utah: Utah State University Extension, 1995), p. 4.

48. Roberta Larson Duyff, *American Dietetic Association's Complete Food & Nutrition Guide,"* p. 146.

49. *Rice, Nutrition and Food Sciences Fact Sheet* (Logan, Utah:

Utah State University Extension), p. 2; see also
www.ext.usu.edu/publica/foodpubs/fn141.pdf

Chapter 9

50. Laura Beil, "Among Major Cancers, Increase in Only One
    Remains a Mystery," *The Dallas Morning News*, September
    27, 1999, p. D7.
51. Lois M. Collins, "Salutary Soy: FDA Says Soy Products
    Provide Health Benefits," *Deseret News*, October 31, 1997
    p. S6

Chapter 10

52. Lori A. Smolin and Mary B. Grosvenor, *Nutrition: Science &
    Applications*, 3d ed. (Orlando, Florida: Harcourt, Inc., 2000),
    pp. 128–60.
53. Ibid.
54. Ibid., p. 143.

Chapter 12

55. Lori A Smolin and Mary B. Grovvenor, *Nutrition*, p. 389.

Chapter 13

56. Vic Sussman, "Muscle Bound," *U.S. News & World Report*,
    May 20, 1991, p. 87.
57. Brigham Young, *Journal of Discourses*, 3:247.

Chapter 14

58. Brigham Young, *Journal of Discourses*, 12:158.
59. Ibid.
60. Brigham Young, *Journal of Discourses*, 4:302.
61. Brigham Young, *Journal of Discourses*, 12:54–55.

62. Brigham Young, *Journal of Discourses*, 12:118; emphasis added.

63. Eric Adler, "Power of Prayer: Religious Appeal Aids Recovery of Patients in Study," *The Salt Lake Tribune*, October 27, 1999, p. A1.

64. Brigham Young, *Journal of Discourses*, 11:329.

65. Brigham Young, *Journal of Discourses*, 12:209.

INDEX